Disability KEY ISSUES AND FUTURE DIRECTIONS

ASSISTIVE TECHNOLOGY
AND SCIENCE

The SAGE Reference Series on Disability: Key Issues and Future Directions

Series Editor: Gary L. Albrecht

Arts and Humanities, by Brenda Jo Brueggemann
Assistive Technology and Science, by Cathy Bodine
Disability Through the Life Course, by Tamar Heller and Sarah Parker Harris
Education, by Cheryl Hanley-Maxwell and Lana Collet-Klingenberg
Employment and Work, by Susanne M. Bruyère and Linda Barrington
Ethics, Law, and Policy, by Jerome E. Bickenbach
Health and Medicine, by Ross M. Mullner
Rehabilitation Interventions, by Margaret A. Turk and Nancy R. Mudrick

Disability KEY ISSUES AND FUTURE DIRECTIONS

ASSISTIVE TECHNOLOGY AND SCIENCE

Cathy Bodine
University of Colorado, Anschutz Medical Campus

SERIES EDITOR
Gary L. Albrecht
University of Illinois at Chicago

⑤SAGE reference

Los Angeles | London | New Delhi
Singapore | Washington DC

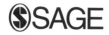

Los Angeles | London | New Delhi
Singapore | Washington DC

FOR INFORMATION:

SAGE Publications, Inc.

2455 Teller Road

Thousand Oaks, California 91320

E-mail: order@sagepub.com

SAGE Publications Ltd.

1 Oliver's Yard

55 City Road

London EC1Y 1SP

United Kingdom

SAGE Publications India Pvt. Ltd.

B 1/I 1 Mohan Cooperative Industrial Area

Mathura Road, New Delhi 110 044

India

SAGE Publications Asia-Pacific Pte. Ltd.

3 Church Street

#10-04 Samsung Hub

Singapore 049483

Publisher: Rolf A. Janke

Acquisitions Editor: Jim Brace-Thompson

Assistant to the Publisher: Michele Thompson

Project Development, Editing, & Management: Kevin Hillstrom,
   Laurie Collier Hillstrom

Production Editor: David C. Felts

Reference Systems Manager: Leticia Gutierrez

Reference Systems Coordinator: Laura Notton

Typesetter: C&M Digitals (P) Ltd.

Proofreader: Stefanie Storholt

Indexer: Ellen Slavitz

Cover Designer: Gail Buschman

Marketing Managers: Kristi Ward, Carmel Schrire

Printed in the United States of America.

Library of Congress Cataloging-in-Publication Data

Bodine, Cathy. Assistive technology and science / Cathy Bodine.

p. cm.—(The SAGE reference series on disability: key issues and future directions)

Includes bibliographical references and index.

ISBN 978-1-4129-8798-1 (cloth)

1. Self-help devices for people with disabilities. I. Title.

HV1569.5.B63 2013
681'.761—dc23   2012035564

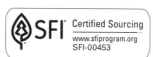

Contents

Series Introduction

The SAGE Reference Series on Disability appears at a time when global attention is being focused on disability at all levels of society. Researchers, service providers, and policymakers are concerned with the prevalence, experience, meanings, and costs of disability because of the growing impact of disability on individuals and their families and subsequent increased demand for services (Banta & de Wit, 2008; Martin et al., 2010; Mont, 2007; Whitaker, 2010). For their part, disabled people and their families are keenly interested in taking a more proactive stance in recognizing and dealing with disability in their lives (Charlton, 1998; Iezzoni & O'Day, 2006). As a result, there is burgeoning literature, heightened Web activity, myriad Internet information and discussion groups, and new policy proposals and programs designed to produce evidence and disseminate information so that people with disabilities may be informed and live more independently (see, for example, the World Institute of Disability Web site at http://www.wid.org, the Center for International Rehabilitation Research Information and Exchange Web site at http://cirrie .buffalo.edu, and the Web portal to caregiver support groups at http:// www.caregiver.com/regionalresources/index.htm).

Disability is recognized as a critical medical and social problem in current society, central to the discussions of health care and social welfare policies taking place around the world. The prominence of these disability issues is highlighted by the attention given to them by the most respected national and international organizations. The *World Report on Disability* (2011), co-sponsored by the World Health Organization (WHO) and the World Bank and based on an analysis of surveys from over 100 countries, estimates that 15% of the world's population (more than 1 billion people) currently experiences disability. This is the best prevalence estimate available today and indicates a marked increase over previous epidemiological calculations. Based on this work, the British medical journal *Lancet* dedicated an entire issue (November 28, 2009) to disability, focusing attention on the salience of the problem for health care systems worldwide. In addition, the WHO has developed community-based rehabilitation principles and strategies which are applicable to communities of diverse cultures and at all levels of development (WHO, 2010). The World Bank is concerned because of the link between disability and poverty (World Bank, 2004). Disability, in their view, could be a major impediment to economic development, particularly in emerging economies.

Efforts to address the problem of disability also have legal and human rights implications. Being disabled has historically led to discrimination, stigma, and dependency, which diminish an individual's full rights to citizenship and equality (European Disability Forum, 2003). In response to these concerns, the United Nations Convention on the Rights of Persons with Disabilities (2008) and the European Union Disability Strategy embodying the Charter of Fundamental Rights (2000) were passed to affirm that disabled people have the right to acquire and change nationalities, cannot be deprived of their ability to exercise liberty, have freedom of movement, are free to leave any country including their own, are not deprived of the right to enter their own country, and have access to the welfare and benefits afforded to any citizen of their country. As of March 31, 2010, 144 nations—including the United States, China, India, and Russia—had signed the U.N. Convention, and the European Union Disability Strategy had been ratified by all members of the European Community. These international agreements supplement and elaborate disability rights legislation such as the Americans with Disabilities Act of 1990 and its amendments, the U.K. Disability Discrimination Act of 1995, and the Disabled Person's Fundamental Law of Japan, revised in 1993.

In the United States, the Institute of Medicine of the National Academy of Sciences has persistently focused attention on the medical, public health, and social policy aspects of disability in a broad-ranging series of reports: *Disability in America* (1991), *Enabling America* (1997), *The Dynamics of Disability: Measuring and Monitoring Disability for Social Security Programs* (2002), *The Future of Disability in America* (2007), and *Improving the Presumptive Disability Decision-Making Process for Veterans* (2008). The Centers for Disease Control have a long-standing interest in diabetes and obesity because of their effects on morbidity, mortality, and disability. Current data show that the incidence and prevalence of obesity is rising across all age groups in the United States, that obesity is related to diabetes, which is also on the rise, and that both, taken together, increase the likelihood of experiencing disability (Bleich et al., 2008; Gill et al., 2010). People with diabetes also are likely to have comorbid depression, which increases their chances of functional disability (Egede, 2004).

Depression and other types of mental illness—like anxiety disorders, alcohol and drug dependence, and impulse-control disorders—are more prevalent than previously thought and often result in disability (Kessler & Wang, 2008). The prevalence of mental disorders in the United States is high, with about half of the population meeting criteria (as measured by the *Diagnostic and Statistical Manual of Mental Disorders,* or DSM-IV) for one or more disorders in their lifetimes, and more than one-quarter of the population meeting criteria for a disorder in any single year. The more severe mental disorders are strongly associated with high comorbidity, resulting in disability.

Major American foundations with significant health portfolios have also turned their attention to disability. The Bill and Melinda Gates Foundation has directed considerable resources to eliminate disability-causing parasitic and communicable diseases such as malaria, elephantiasis, and river blindness. These efforts are designed to prevent and control disability-causing conditions in the developing world that inhibit personal independence and economic development. The Robert Wood Johnson Foundation has a long-standing program on self-determination for people with developmental disabilities in the United States aimed at increasing their ability to participate fully in society, and the Hogg Foundation is dedicated to improving mental health awareness and services. Taken in concert, these activities underscore the recognized importance of disability in the present world.

Disability Concepts, Models, and Theories

There is an immense literature on disability concepts, models, and theories. An in-depth look at these issues and controversies can be found in the *Handbook of Disability Studies* (Albrecht, Seelman, & Bury, 2001), in the *Encyclopedia of Disability* (Albrecht, 2006), and in "The Sociology of Disability: Historical Foundations and Future Directions" (Albrecht, 2010). For the purposes of this reference series, it is useful to know that the World Health Organization, in the International Classification of Functioning, Disability and Health (ICF), defines disability as "an umbrella term for impairments, activity limitations or participation restrictions" (WHO, 2001, p. 3). ICF also lists environmental factors that interact with all these constructs. Further, the WHO defines impairments as "problems in body function or structure such as significant deviation or loss"; activity limitations as "difficulties an individual may have in executing activities"; participation as "involvement in a life situation"; and environmental factors as those components of "the physical, social and attitudinal environment in which people live and conduct their lives" (WHO, 2001, p. 10). The U.N. Convention on the Rights of Persons with Disabilities, in turn, defines disability as including "those who have long-term physical, mental, intellectual or sensory impairments which in interaction with various barriers may hinder their full and effective participation in society on an equal basis with others." In the introduction to the *Lancet* special issue on disability, Officer and Groce (2009) conclude that "both the ICF and the Convention view disability as the outcome of complex interactions between health conditions and features of an individual's physical, social, and attitudinal environment that hinder their full and effective participation in society" (p. 1795). Hence, disability scholars and activists alike are concerned with breaking down physical, environmental, economic, and social barriers so that disabled people can live independently and participate as fully as possible in society.

Types of Disability

Interest in disability by medical practitioners has traditionally been condition specific (such as spinal cord injury or disabilities due to heart disease), reflecting the medical model approach to training and disease taxonomies. Similarly, disabled people and their families are often most concerned about their particular conditions and how best to deal with them. The SAGE Reference Series on Disability recognizes that there are a broad range of disabilities that can be generally conceived of as falling in the categories of physical, mental, intellectual, and sensory disabilities. In practice, disabled persons may have more than one disability and are often difficult to place in one disability category. For instance, a spinal-cord injured individual might experience depression, and a person with multiple sclerosis may simultaneously deal with physical and sensory disabilities. It is also important to note that disabilities are dynamic. People do experience different rates of onset, progression, remission, and even transition from being disabled at one point in time, to not being disabled at another, to being disabled again. Examples of this change in disability status include disability due to bouts of arthritis, Guillain-Barré Syndrome, and postpartum depression.

Disability Language

The symbols and language used to represent disability have sparked contentious debates over the years. In the *Handbook of Disability Studies* (Albrecht, Seelman, & Bury, 2001) and the *Encyclopedia of Disability* (Albrecht, 2006), authors from different countries were encouraged to use the terms and language of their cultures, but to explain them when necessary. In the present volumes, authors may use "people with disabilities" or "disabled people" to refer to individuals experiencing disability. Scholars in the United States have preferred "people with disabilities" (people-first language), while those in the United Kingdom, Canada, and Australia generally use "disabled people." In languages other than English, scholars typically use some form of the "disabled people" idiom. The U.S. version emphasizes American exceptionalism and the individual, whereas "disabled people" highlights the group and their minority status or state of being different. In my own writing, I have chosen "disabled people" because it stresses human diversity and variation.

In a recent discussion of this issue, DePoy and Gilson (2010) "suggest that maintaining debate and argument on what language is most correct derails a larger and more profound needed change, that of equalizing resources, valuation, and respect. Moreover, . . . locating disability 'with a person' reifies its embodiment and flies in the very face of the social model that person-first language is purported to espouse. . . . We have not heard anyone suggest that beauty, kindness, or even unkindness be located after personhood." While the debate is not likely over, we state why we use the language that we do.

Organization of the Series

These issues were important in conceiving of and organizing the SAGE Reference Series on Disability. Instead of developing the series around specific disabilities resulting from Parkinson's disease or bi-polar disorder, or according to the larger categories of physical, mental, intellectual, and sensory disabilities, we decided to concentrate on the major topics that confront anyone interested in or experiencing disability. Thus, the series consists of eight volumes constructed around the following topics:

- Arts and Humanities
- Assistive Technology and Science

- Disability Through the Life Course
- Education
- Employment and Work
- Ethics, Law, and Policy
- Health and Medicine
- Rehabilitation Interventions

To provide structure, we chose to use a similar organization for each volume. Therefore, each volume contains the following elements:

Series Introduction

Preface

About the Author

About the Series Editor

Chapter 1. Introduction, Background, and History

Chapter 2. Current Issues, Controversies, and Solutions

Chapter 3. Chronology of Critical Events

Chapter 4. Biographies of Key Contributors in the Field

Chapter 5. Annotated Data, Statistics, Tables, and Graphs

Chapter 6. Annotated List of Organizations and Associations

Chapter 7. Selected Print and Electronic Resources

Glossary of Key Terms

Index

The Audience

The eight-volume SAGE Reference Series on Disability targets an audience of undergraduate students and general readers that uses both academic and public libraries. However, the content and depth of the series will also make it attractive to graduate students, researchers, and policymakers. The series has been edited to have a consistent format and accessible style. The focus in each volume is on providing lay-friendly overviews of broad issues and guideposts for further research and exploration.

The series is innovative in that it will be published and marketed worldwide, with each volume available in electronic format soon after it appears in print. The print version consists of eight bound volumes. The electronic version is available through the SAGE Reference Online platform, which hosts 200 handbooks and encyclopedias across the social sciences, including the *Handbook of Disability Studies* and the *Encyclopedia of Disability*. With access to this platform through college, university, and public libraries, students, the lay public, and scholars can search these interrelated disability and social science sources from their computers or handheld and smart phone devices. The movement to an electronic platform presages the cloud computing revolution coming upon us. Cloud computing "refers to 'everything' a user may reach via the Internet, including services, storage, applications and people" (Hoehl & Sieh, 2010). According to Ray Ozzie (2010), recently Microsoft's chief architect, "We're moving toward a world of (1) cloud-based continuous services that connect us all and do our bidding, and (2) appliance-like connected devices enabling us to interact with those cloud-based services." Literally, information will be available at consumers' fingertips. Given the ample links to other resources in emerging databases, they can pursue any topic of interest in detail. This resource builds on the massive efforts to make information available to decision makers in real time, such as computerizing health and hospital records so that the diagnosis and treatment of chronic diseases and disabilities can be better managed (Celler, Lovell, & Basilakis, 2003). The SAGE Reference Series on Disability provides Internet and Web site addresses which lead the user into a world of social networks clustered around disability in general and specific conditions and issues. Entering and engaging with social networks revolving around health and disability promises to help individuals make more informed decisions and provide support in times of need (Smith & Christakis, 2008). The SAGE Reference Online platform will also be configured and updated to make it increasingly accessible to disabled people.

The SAGE Reference Series on Disability provides an extensive index for each volume. Through its placement on the SAGE Reference Online platform, the series will be fully searchable and cross-referenced, will allow keyword searching, and will be connected to the *Handbook of Disability Studies* and the *Encyclopedia of Disability*.

The authors of the volumes have taken considerable effort to vet the references, data, and resources for accuracy and credibility. The multiple Web sites for current data, information, government and United Nations documents, research findings, expert recommendations, self-help, discussion groups, and social policy are particularly useful, as they are being continuously updated. Examples of current and forthcoming data are the results and analysis of the findings of the U.S. 2010 Census, the ongoing reports of the Centers for Disease Control on disability, the World Health Organization's *World Report on Disability* and its updates, the World Bank reports on disability, poverty, and development, and reports from major foundations like Robert Wood Johnson, Bill and Melinda Gates, Ford, and Hogg. In terms of clinical outcomes, the evaluation of cost-effective interventions, management of disability, and programs that work, enormous attention is being given to evidence-based outcomes (Brownson, Fielding, & Maylahn, 2009; Marcus et al., 2006; Wolinsky et al., 2007) and comparative effectiveness research (Etheredge, 2010; Inglehart, 2010). Such data force a re-examination of policymakers' arguments. For example, there is mounting evidence that demonstrates the beneficial effects of exercise on preventing disability and enhancing function (Marcus et al., 2006). Recent studies also show that some health care reform initiatives may negatively affect disabled people's access to and costs of health care (Burns, Shah, & Smith, 2010). Furthermore, the seemingly inexorable rise in health care spending may not be correlated with desirable health outcomes (Rothberg et al., 2010). In this environment, valid data are the currency of the discussion (Andersen, Lollar, & Meyers, 2000). The authors' hopes are that this reference series will encourage students and the lay public to base their discussions and decisions on valid outcome data. Such an approach tempers the influence of ideologies surrounding health care and misconceptions about disabled people, their lives, and experiences.

SAGE Publications has made considerable effort to make these volumes accessible to disabled people in the printed book version and in the electronic platform format. In turn, SAGE and other publishers and vendors like Amazon are incorporating greater flexibility in the user interface to improve functionality to a broad range of users, such as disabled people. These efforts are important for disabled people as universities, governments, and health service delivery organizations are moving toward a paperless environment.

In the spirit of informed discussion and transparency, may this reference series encourage people from many different walks of life to become knowledgeable and engaged in the disability world. As a consequence, social policies should become better informed and individuals and families should be able to make better decisions regarding the experience of disability in their lives.

Acknowledgments

I would like to recognize the vision of Rolf Janke in developing SAGE Publications' presence in the disability field, as represented by the *Handbook of Disability Studies* (2001), the five-volume *Encyclopedia of Disability* (2006), and now the eight-volume SAGE Reference Series on Disability. These products have helped advance the field and have made critical work accessible to scholars, students, and the general public through books and now the SAGE Reference Online platform. Jim Brace-Thompson at SAGE handled the signing of contracts and kept this complex project coordinated and moving on time. Kevin Hillstrom and Laurie Collier Hillstrom at Northern Lights Writers Group were intrepid in taking the composite pieces of this project and polishing and editing them into a coherent whole that is approachable, consistent in style and form, and rich in content. The authors of the eight volumes—Linda Barrington, Jerome Bickenbach, Cathy Bodine, Brenda Brueggemann, Susanne Bruyère, Lana Collet-Klingenberg, Cheryl Hanley-Maxwell, Sarah Parker Harris, Tamar Heller, Nancy Mudrick, Ross Mullner, and Peggy Turk—are to be commended for their enthusiasm, creativity, and fortitude in delivering high-quality volumes on a tight deadline. I was fortunate to work with such accomplished scholars.

Discussions with Barbara Altman, Colin Barnes, Catherine Barral, Len Barton, Isabelle Baszanger, Peter Blanck, Mary Boulton, David Braddock, Richard Burkhauser, Mike Bury, Ann Caldwell, Lennard Davis, Patrick Devlieger, Ray Fitzpatrick, Lawrence Frey, Carol Gill, Tamar Heller, Gary Kielhofner, Soewarta Kosen, Jo Lebeer, Mitch Loeb, Don Lollar, Paul Longmore, Ros Madden, Maria Martinho, Dennis Mathews, Sophie Mitra, Daniel Mont, Alana Officer, Randall Parker, David Pfeiffer, Jean-François Raveau, James Rimmer, Ed Roberts, Jean-Marie Robine, Joan Rogers, Richard Scotch, Kate Seelman, Tom Shakespeare, Sandor Sipos, Henri-Jacques Stiker, Edna Szymanski, Jutta Traviranus, Bryan Turner, Greg Vanderheiden, Isabelle Ville, Larry Voss, Ann Waldschmidt, and Irving Kenneth Zola over the years contributed to the content, logic, and structure of the series. They also were a wonderful source of suggestions for authors.

I would also like to acknowledge the hospitality and support of the Belgian Academy of Science and the Arts, the University of Leuven, Nuffield College, the University of Oxford, the Fondation Maison des Sciences de l'Homme, Paris, and the Department of Disability and Human

Development at the University of Illinois at Chicago, who provided the time and environments to conceive of and develop the project. While none of these people or institutions is responsible for any deficiencies in the work, they all helped enormously in making it better.

Gary L. Albrecht
University of Illinois at Chicago
University of Leuven
Belgian Academy of Science and Arts

References

Albrecht, G. L. (Ed.). (2006). *Encyclopedia of disability* (5 vols.). Thousand Oaks, CA: Sage.

Albrecht, G. L. (2010). The sociology of disability: Historical foundations and future directions. In C. Bird, A. Fremont, S. Timmermans, & P. Conrad (Eds.), *Handbook of medical sociology* (6th ed., pp. 192–209). Nashville, TN: Vanderbilt University Press.

Albrecht, G. L., Seelman, K. D., & Bury, M. (Eds.). (2001). *Handbook of disability studies.* Thousand Oaks, CA: Sage.

Andersen, E. M., Lollar, D. J., & Meyers, A. R. (2000). Disability outcomes research: Why this supplement, on this topic, at this time? *Archives of Physical Medicine and Rehabilitation, 81,* S1–S4.

Banta, H. D., & de Wit, G. A. (2008). Public health services and cost-effectiveness analysis. *Annual Review of Public Health, 29,* 383–397.

Bleich, S., Cutler, D., Murray, C., & Adams, A. (2008). Why is the developed world obese? *Annual Review of Public Health, 29,* 273–295.

Brownson, R. C., Fielding, J. E., & Maylahn, C. M. (2009). Evidence-based public health: A fundamental concept for public health practice. *Annual Review of Public Health, 30,* 175–201.

Burns, M., Shah, N., & Smith, M. (2010). Why some disabled adults in Medicaid face large out-of-pocket expenses. *Health Affairs, 29,* 1517–1522.

Celler, B. G., Lovell, N. H., & Basilakis, J. (2003). Using information technology to improve the management of chronic disease. *Medical Journal of Australia, 179,* 242–246.

Charlton, J. I. (1998). *Nothing about us without us: Disability, oppression and empowerment.* Berkeley: University of California Press.

DePoy, E., & Gilson, S. F. (2010). *Studying disability: Multiple theories and responses.* Thousand Oaks, CA: Sage.

Egede, L. E. (2004). Diabetes, major depression, and functional disability among U.S. adults. *Diabetes Care, 27,* 421–428.

Etheredge, L. M. (2010). Creating a high-performance system for comparative effectiveness research. *Health Affairs, 29,* 1761–1767.

European Disability Forum. (2003). *Disability and social exclusion in the European Union: Time for change, tools for change.* Athens: Greek National Confederation of Disabled People.

European Union. (2000). *Charter of fundamental rights.* Retrieved from http://www.europarll.europa.eu/charter

Gill, T. M., Gahbauer, E. A., Han, L., & Allore, H. G. (2010). Trajectories of disability in the last year of life. *The New England Journal of Medicine, 362*(13), 1173–1180.

Hoehl, A. A., & Sieh, K. A. (2010). *Cloud computing and disability communities: How can cloud computing support a more accessible information age and society?* Boulder, CO: Coleman Institute.

Iezzoni, L. I., & O'Day, B. L. (2006). *More than ramps.* Oxford, UK: Oxford University Press.

Inglehart, J. K. (2010). The political fight over comparative effectiveness research. *Health Affairs, 29,* 1757–1760.

Institute of Medicine. (1991). *Disability in America.* Washington, DC: National Academies Press.

Institute of Medicine. (1997). *Enabling America.* Washington, DC: National Academies Press.

Institute of Medicine. (2001). *Health and behavior: The interplay of biological, behavioral and societal influences.* Washington, DC: National Academies Press.

Institute of Medicine. (2002). *The dynamics of disability: Measuring and monitoring disability for social security programs.* Washington, DC: National Academies Press.

Institute of Medicine. (2007). *The future of disability in America.* Washington, DC: National Academies Press.

Institute of Medicine. (2008). *Improving the presumptive disability decision-making process for veterans.* Washington, DC: National Academies Press.

Kessler, R. C., & Wang, P. S. (2008). The descriptive epidemiology of commonly occurring mental disorders in the United States. *Annual Review of Public Health, 29,* 115–129.

Marcus, B. H., Williams, D. M., Dubbert, P. M., Sallis, J. F., King, A. C., Yancey, A. K., et al. (2006). Physical activity intervention studies. *Circulation, 114,* 2739–2752.

Martin, L. G., Freedman, V. A., Schoeni, R. F., & Andreski, P. M. (2010). Trends in disability and related chronic conditions among people ages 50 to 64. *Health Affairs, 29*(4), 725–731.

Mont, D. (2007). *Measuring disability prevalence* (World Bank working paper). Washington, DC: The World Bank.

Officer, A., & Groce, N. E. (2009). Key concepts in disability. *The Lancet, 374,* 1795–1796.

Ozzie, R. (2010, October 28). *Dawn of a new day.* Ray Ozzie's Blog. Retrieved from http://ozzie.net/docs/dawn-of-a-new-day

Rothberg, M. B., Cohen, J., Lindenauer, P., Masetti, J., & Auerbach, A. (2010). Little evidence of correlation between growth in health care spending and reduced mortality. *Health Affairs, 29,* 1523–1531.

Smith, K. P., & Christakis, N. A. (2008). Social networks and health. *Annual Review of Sociology, 34*, 405–429.

United Nations. (2008). *Convention on the rights of persons with disabilities.* New York: United Nations. Retrieved from http://un.org/disabilities/convention

Whitaker, R. T. (2010). *Anatomy of an epidemic: Magic bullets, psychiatric drugs, and the astonishing rise of mental illness in America.* New York: Crown.

Wolinsky, F. D., Miller, D. K., Andresen, E. M., Malmstrom, T. K., Miller, J. P., & Miller, T. R. (2007). Effect of subclinical status in functional limitation and disability on adverse health outcomes 3 years later. *The Journals of Gerontology: Series A, 62*, 101–106.

World Bank Disability and Development Team. (2004). *Poverty reduction strategies: Their importance for disability.* Washington, DC: World Bank.

World Health Organization. (2001). *International classification of functioning, disability and health.* Geneva: Author.

World Health Organization. (2010). *Community-based rehabilitation guidelines.* Geneva and Washington, DC: Author.

World Health Organization, & World Bank. (2011). *World report on disability.* Geneva: World Health Organization.

Preface

In today's world, technology has become ubiquitous. Cell phones, tablets, desktops, ATMs, games, and cash registers are all connected. For people with disabilities, technology not only creates access to the world at large, it also creates greater opportunities for education, work, and play. On the flip side, technology *can* make life more difficult for persons with disabilities. Small buttons and keyboards that are confusing, graphics without tag lines to tell the individual what is on the screen, and many other technical aspects can create confusion, frustration, and limited access to the world at large. But these are all aspects that can be dealt with.

This volume explores the history and current status of assistive technology (AT) and accessible mainstream commercial technologies. Its purpose is to share where we are in the life cycle of technology for persons with disabilities; to examine historical aspects and future trends, along with legislative and funding issues. The need for professional development training and outreach to create an informed constituency is also explored. This volume introduces the topic of assistive technology and offers resources and information about where to go to learn more.

In Chapter 1, *Introduction, Background, and History,* we provide a brief overview of the field of assistive technology, which includes both devices *and* services. This overview of AT devices and services includes definitions, history, and legislation. It discusses the types of AT available for people with communication disorders, impaired mobility, hearing and visual impairments, and cognitive/learning disabilities. It also describes the selection of appropriate technology and training in its use, suggests ways to avoid the abandonment of assistive technology by clients and caregivers, and discusses the principles of clinical assessment and physician responsibility. Finally, it briefly discusses the future in terms of research and development and application of emerging technologies to the needs of people with disabilities.

In Chapter 2, *Current Issues, Controversies, and Solutions,* we discuss the issues that surround the field of AT. Even though AT devices and services have existed for many years, the actual *field* of assistive technology is still emerging. While substantial progress has also been made in developing thousands of assistive technologies and creating enhanced accessibility for persons with disabilities to mainstream commercial products such as computers and cell phones, obtaining funding for these devices and services remains an often-insurmountable barrier. This chapter discusses issues that arise for an often-underserved population as a result of the topsy-turvy growth of the field along with the exponential explosion of new and emerging technologies.

In Chapter 3, *Chronology of Critical Events,* we explore, beginning in 1808, the history of technology developments and applications for persons with disabilities, as well as legislation, public policies, and civil rights movements related to persons with disabilities. We hope that the reader will see the trends and conditions that have impacted the rights and responsibilities of persons with disabilities, their families, care providers, and AT manufacturers and developers.

In Chapter 4, *Biographies of Key Contributors in the Field,* we provide information on a number of amazing individuals with disabilities, policymakers, developers, and caregivers who have been influential in furthering the field of AT for people with disabilities. Authors and advocates of important public policies and legislation addressing the benefits and risks of using technology to increase independence for persons with disabilities are also highlighted. Biographical sketches are included for each person and references for more information are provided.

In Chapter 5, *Annotated Data, Statistics, Tables, and Graphs,* we provide information on technology and disability to the extent possible. This was a difficult chapter to prepare, as the field of assistive technology suffers from a paucity of available data. This chapter may, in the end, be the most important, as it so clearly delineates what data is available and the age of the data. Although much of the data felt too old to include, it was not superseded by new information. This chapter also, more than any other chapter within the book, points the reader to the critical need to develop strategic and comprehensive data collection systems in order for us to truly analyze where we are and where we need to go in terms of evidence-based outcomes, usage data, and much more.

Chapter 6, *Annotated List of Organizations and Associations,* and Chapter 7, *Selected Print and Electronic Resources,* include reference material in order for the reader to seek out more information and available research on selected topics. In these chapters, we provide a brief description, contact information, and Web sites for multiple organizations and associations, as well as annotated listings of print and electronic resources. The topic areas are wide ranging and, we hope, of much use for the reader.

The goal of this volume is to excite next-generation researchers, people with disabilities, and their caregivers and family members who may be new, or relatively new, to the potential that technology has to offer for persons with disabilities. Technology applicable to persons with disabilities is becoming, and will become, ever more recognizable as a first-line option for persons with disabilities who wish, just like persons without disabilities, to go about their lives as productive and independent citizens.

Acknowledgments

An effort such as this volume in the Sage Reference Series on Disability would not have been possible without the support and efforts of the series editor, Gary Albrecht, and Jim Brace-Thompson, senior editor at Sage Reference. Kevin Hillstrom and Laurie Collier Hillstrom of Northern Lights Writers Group were unbelievably kind and supportive during the often-frustrating task of pushing the author and our contributors to an end product. They all deserve a very large gold star!

This volume could not have been completed without the able contributions of faculty at Assistive Technology Partners, Departments of Physical Medicine and Rehabilitation, Pediatrics and Bioengineering, University of Colorado, School of Medicine.

Lorrie Harkness, Ph.D., and Maureen Melonis, MNS, CCC-SLP, faculty with extraordinary experience and knowledge within the field of AT, provided immense support and help in the preparation of this volume. Dr. Harkness contributed extensively to Chapter 3, *Chronology of Critical Events* and Chapter 6, *Annotated List of Organizations and Associations*. She deserves full credit for her attention to detail and writing ability. Ms. Melonis also contributed to Chapter 3 and particularly to Chapter 7: *Print and Electronic Resources*. Both Dr. Harkness and Ms. Melonis were instrumental in completing Chapter 4, *Biographies of Key Contributors in the Field*, and Chapter 5, *Annotated Data, Statistics, Tables, and Graphs*. Without their work, this volume could not have been completed. Their contribution to this volume enabled us to provide the reader with as much historical and current data as possible. It is not often that the word *team* can be used when describing a long and arduous process. In this case, the word *team* amply describes what we are about at Assistive Technology Partners.

Without these terrific partners and friends, this volume would not have been possible, and I am forever thankful for their help and support.

Cathy Bodine

About the Author

Cathy Bodine, Ph.D., CCC-SLP, is an Associate Professor and Section Head in the Department of Physical Medicine and Rehabilitation and Department of Pediatrics, an Affiliate Faculty Member in the Department of Bioengineering, and Executive Director of Assistive Technology Partners at the University of Colorado, Anschutz Medical Campus.

Dr. Bodine began her career in assistive technology in 1985. She joined the faculty of the University of Colorado, Anschutz Medical Campus in 1996. Today, she is internationally recognized for her leadership in the field of assistive technology and vigorously pursues her passions for new product design, research, service to families and persons with disabilities, and the professional assistive technology community at large through her leadership of Assistive Technology Partners.

Dr. Bodine has served as the principal investigator (PI) for a number of preservice professional preparation grants, as well as the Colorado Assistive Technology Act. In addition, she has served as the PI for several research and development projects leading to new designs in AT devices. She also led a U.S. Department of Education funded Field Initiated Development Project utilizing the *International Classification of Functioning* to measure assistive technology outcomes. She is the principal investigator for the Rehabilitation Engineering Research Center for Advancing Cognitive Technologies (RERC-ACT). Dr. Bodine serves on numerous national and international boards and is a frequent author and lecturer.

About the
Series Editor

Gary L. Albrecht is a Fellow of the Royal Belgian Academy of Arts and Sciences, Extraordinary Guest Professor of Social Sciences, University of Leuven, Belgium, and Professor Emeritus of Public Health and of Disability and Human Development at the University of Illinois at Chicago. After receiving his Ph.D. from Emory University, he has served on the faculties of Emory University in Sociology and Psychiatry, Northwestern University in Sociology, Rehabilitation Medicine, and the Kellogg School of Management, and the University of Illinois at Chicago (UIC) in the School of Public Health and in the Department of Disability and Human Development. Since retiring from the UIC in 2005, he has divided his time between Europe and the United States, working in Brussels, Belgium, and Boulder, Colorado. He has served as a Scholar in Residence at the Maison des Sciences de l'Homme (MSH) in Paris, a visiting Fellow at Nuffield College, the University of Oxford, and a Fellow in Residence at the Royal Flemish Academy of Science and Arts, Brussels.

His research has focused on how adults acknowledge, interpret, and respond to unanticipated life events, such as disability onset. His work, supported by over $25 million of funding, has resulted in 16 books and over 140 articles and book chapters. He is currently working on a longitudinal study of disabled Iranian, Moroccan, Turkish, Jewish, and Congolese immigrants to Belgium. Another current project involves working with an international team on "Disability: A Global Picture," Chapter 2 of the *World Report on Disability*, co-sponsored by the World Health Organization and the World Bank, published in 2011.

He is past Chair of the Medical Sociology Section of the American Sociological Association, a past member of the Executive Committee of the

Disability Forum of the American Public Health Association, an early member of the Society for Disability Studies, and an elected member of the Society for Research in Rehabilitation (UK). He has received the Award for the Promotion of Human Welfare and the Eliot Freidson Award for the book *The Disability Business: Rehabilitation in America*. He also has received a Switzer Distinguished Research Fellowship, Schmidt Fellowship, New York State Supreme Court Fellowship, Kellogg Fellowship, National Library of Medicine Fellowship, World Health Organization Fellowship, the Lee Founders Award from the Society for the Study of Social Problems, the Licht Award from the American Congress of Rehabilitation Medicine, the University of Illinois at Chicago Award for Excellence in Teaching, and has been elected Fellow of the American Association for the Advancement of Science (AAAS). He has led scientific delegations in rehabilitation medicine to the Soviet Union and the People's Republic of China and served on study sections, grant review panels, and strategic planning committees on disability in Australia, Canada, the European Community, France, Ireland, Japan, Poland, South Africa, Sweden, the United Kingdom, the United States, and the World Health Organization, Geneva. His most recent books are *The Handbook of Social Studies in Health and Medicine*, edited with Ray Fitzpatrick and Susan Scrimshaw (SAGE, 2000), the *Handbook of Disability Studies*, edited with Katherine D. Seelman and Michael Bury (SAGE, 2001), and the five-volume *Encyclopedia of Disability* (SAGE, 2006).

One

Introduction, Background, and History

Introduction

This chapter provides an overview of assistive technology (AT) devices and services, including definitions, history, and legislation. It also discusses the use of assistive technology for people with communication disorders, impaired mobility, hearing and visual impairments, and cognitive/learning disabilities. It describes the selection of appropriate technology and training in its use, suggests ways to avoid the abandonment of assistive technology by clients and caregivers, and discusses the principles of clinical assessment and physician responsibility. Finally, it briefly discusses the future in terms of research and development and application of emerging technologies to the needs of people with disabilities.

What Is Assistive Technology?

In the United States, a legal definition of assistive technology was first published in the Technology-Related Assistance for Individuals with Disabilities Act of 1988 and remains in effect today via Public Law 100–407.

Any item, piece of equipment, or system, whether acquired commercially, modified, or customized, that is commonly used to increase, maintain, or improve functional capabilities of individuals with disabilities.

This definition also includes a second component defining assistive technology services as "Any service that directly assists an individual with a disability in the selection, acquisition, or use of an assistive technology device." P.L. 100–407 specified the following assistive technology services:

- Evaluating an individual with a disability in terms of their goals, needs, and functional abilities in his or her customary environment;
- Purchasing, leasing, or otherwise providing for the acquisition of assistive technology by persons with disabilities;
- Selecting, designing, fitting, customizing, adapting, applying, retaining, repairing, or replacing assistive technology devices;
- Coordinating and using other therapies, interventions, or services with assistive technology devices, such as those associated with existing education and rehabilitation plans and programs;
- Training or technical assistance for the person with a disability or, if appropriate, his or her family; and
- Training or technical assistance for professionals (including individuals providing education or rehabilitation services), employers, or other individuals who provide services to, employ, or are otherwise substantially involved in the major life functions of children with disabilities (King, 1999).

Since 1988 this definition has also been used in other U.S. Federal legislation authorizing services or supports for persons with disabilities. The Individuals with Disabilities Education Act (IDEA) and Reauthorization of the Rehabilitation Act are both examples of legislation that further codifies P.L. 100–407.

So what is AT? In short, AT is *a tool* used by someone with a disability to perform everyday tasks, such as getting dressed, moving around, or controlling his or her environment, learning, working, or engaging in recreational activities. Less than 30 years ago, there were fewer than 100 assistive devices commercially available. Today, more than 30,000 assistive devices are listed on the AbleData Web site (www.abledata.com). AT use often begins as early as birth and continues throughout the life span of individuals with disabilities.

Assistive technology devices are designed to facilitate functional abilities and to meet the needs of humans throughout their varied life stages and roles. ATs have been designed that target the sensory impairments (vision, hearing, touch); motor impairments of both upper and lower body (walking, moving, using hands and arms); communication impairments (ranging from poor speech articulation or dysarthria to devices that speak for persons who are completely nonverbal); as well as cognitive impairments.

During our lifetime, at least one in five persons living in the United States will experience a disabling condition and could benefit from the use of AT devices and/or services. Each of us will also experience something known as situationally induced disability. An example of a situationally induced disability might be found in a work environment that is so loud that workers are unable to hear each other (hearing impairment), or it might occur as a result of going without enough sleep (cognitive/sensory impairments). In many cases, ATs can be used to improve transitory instances of disabilities. In a loud environment, electronic texting might be used to compensate for the loss of hearing. When someone is sleepy, built-in sensors in cars are now available to help persons remain alert and safe. As technologies continue to become more powerful and easier to use, more and more citizens can and will benefit from their use.

It is important to remember that assistive technology device usage and requirements can change over time as individuals mature and assume different life roles. For example, toddlers' needs change dramatically when they are old enough to attend preschool or kindergarten. Young adults who are leaving high school to enter the workforce or move on to college may also experience significant changes in their technology needs. Seniors who would like to age in place may experience significant changes in their motor, cognitive, and sensory systems and can benefit immensely from the proper application of ATs.

AT needs and usage can also change when someone has a degenerative disorder such as multiple sclerosis (MS), amyotrophic lateral sclerosis (ALS; also known as Lou Gehrig's disease), or any of the dementias (Alzheimer's disease, Parkinson's disease, etc.). Consequently, there is no "one size fits all" technology available.

History of AT

Humans have used tools to complete everyday tasks throughout history. However, the use of technology as a tool for persons with disabilities is often viewed as something that has just emerged in the past two or three decades. Interestingly, James and Thorpe (1994) describe any number of assistive devices used as early as the sixth or seventh century B.C.

Their descriptions include partial dentures, artificial legs and hands, and drinking tubes or straws. The earliest documented account of optical and lens technologies, or eyeglasses, came from Venice around A.D. 1300 (King, 1999). Use of the term *assistive technology* (AT) to describe devices used to facilitate the accomplishment of everyday tasks by persons with disabilities is actually the more recent development.

Chapter 3: Chronology of Events highlights the emergence of technologies with a direct impact on the history of AT for disability. However, there have been several key transitions and world incidents over the centuries that have had a direct impact on the development of technologies to support persons with disabilities. For example, crutches and canes have been around for literally thousands of years as mobility assisting devices. Other than changes in the material composition (wood to metal) and some adaptations for comfort, very little has actually changed in terms of the purpose and overall style of these mobility aids. In developing countries today, canes and crutches are still designed from locally available materials and, in many cases, mimic the design of those found in ancient Rome.

Wars have always had a direct impact on the development of ATs and other medical advances over the centuries. In the United States, the Civil War led to major advancements in prosthetic limb development. In 1863, Dubois Parmelee developed the first socket with a suction attachment, significantly improving the fit and function of lower-limb prosthetics (Murphy, Cook, & Harvey, 1982). Although the materials used today represent huge improvements in terms of durability and comfort, his essential design remains in use. During World War II, significant advancements in orthopedic devices and services continued. Recent conflicts in Iraq and Afghanistan have led to new and exciting leaps forward in prosthetics. Today's prosthetics are lighter, more flexible in terms of foot and hand function, and are often driven by advanced microprocessor chips (Weires, 2008).

The advent of the computer, with the microprocessor electronic circuit chip, has arguably had the biggest impact on the advancement of assistive technologies in the past 25 years. Assistive software for learning, literacy development, and reading of text out loud for those who cannot see or cannot read, along with communication devices that speak for individuals who are nonverbal, have all benefited from this single advancement.

Since World War II, wheelchairs have also benefited from significant revisions in overall design for comfort, durability, and weight. Today's high-tech wheelchairs incorporate sophisticated computer-based electronics and can be driven using head controls, single switches attached near any muscle that is capable of triggering a response, and even a "sip-n-puff" straw.

Hearing aids were first patented in the 1890s. Today's hearing aids bear little resemblance to the bulky, body-worn devices of the past. Hearing aids have been miniaturized, can now be easily worn inside the ear canal, and are powered by advanced microelectronics. Mimicking functions of the central nervous system, hearing aids today have the ability to filter extraneous or loud noises, enabling comfort and more functional usage by wearers.

Beginning in World War II and continuing well through Vietnam, hearing damage has been a leading disability for the military. Large numbers of soldiers caught in roadside bombings and firefights in Iraq and Afghanistan are returning to the United States with permanent hearing loss and tinnitus or "ringing in the ears." Nearly 70,000 of the more than 1.3 million troops who have served in the two war zones are collecting disability for tinnitus, a potentially debilitating ringing in the ears, and more than 58,000 are already qualified for disability services for hearing loss. A primary cause of this hearing loss is the use of powerful roadside bombs. The concussion caused by these blasts is significant enough to rupture eardrums and break the small bones located inside the ear. The military has been working to develop better and easier-to-use earplugs, troop education about hearing protection, and on-site testing in the field to identify hearing loss or injury more quickly. The military is also supporting the development and advancement of new technologies to aid soldiers with tinnitus and/or hearing loss.

Another side effect of the current conflict is the increasing number of soldiers returning with mild to profound cognitive impairments. Tremendous efforts are underway to develop technologies to aid in the rehabilitation of these deficits as well as to facilitate re-entry into the soldiers' home communities. A number of federally funded initiatives are underway to develop prompting technologies for individuals struggling with memory impairments. Technologies are being developed to aid those who cannot remember what step needs to happen next; cognitive aids for taking medications on time; and other technologies to support basic activities of daily living, such as hygiene, meal preparation, and recreational activities.

Robotic technologies are also beginning to have an impact on rehabilitation treatment and to be used for assistance at home and in the community for individuals with a variety of disabilities. The success of robots in rehabilitation has been driven by their capacity to control the position and forces applied to limbs, and their inherent ability to easily, objectively, and reliably quantify sensorimotor behavior (Kawamura & Iskarous, 1994; Lathan & Malley, 2001; Lieberman & Breazeal, 2007; Marchal-Crespo & Rienkensmeyer, 2008; Mataric et al., 2007; Thrun, 2002; Turkle, 2006). Robotic technologies are ideally suited for clinically assessing sensory, motor, and cognitive impairments in stroke and other neurological disorders, including traumatic brain injury. With the worldwide shift in demographics to an aging society, countries in Europe, Asia, and North America in particular are researching how robotics devices and tools can be used as assistive devices to aid seniors who wish to remain at home; support caregivers in completing medical tasks, such as reporting vital signs; help seniors to complete exercise activities; and alert family members or health care workers when there seems to be a problem.

Assistive Technology and the International Classification of Functioning (ICF)

The term *disability* is not always precise and quantifiable. Further, the concept of disability is not even agreed upon by persons who self-identify as having a disability, by professionals who study disability, or by the general public (Bodine, 2009). This lack of agreement creates an obstacle to the study of disability and to the fair and effective administration of programs and policies intended for people with disabilities (Brown, 2008). With this issue in mind, the World Health Organization (WHO) developed a global common health language—one that includes physical, mental, and social well-being. The International Classification of Impairment, Disabilities, and Handicaps (ICIDH) was first published by the WHO in 1980 as a tool for classification of the "consequences of disease." The newest version, *International Classification of Functioning, Disability, and Health* (ICF), moves away from a "consequence of disease" classification (1980 version) to a more positive "components of health" classification. This latest version provides a common framework and language for the description of health and health-related domains and uses the following definitions:

- Body functions are the physiological functions of body systems (including psychological functions).
- Body structures are anatomical parts of the body, such as organs, limbs, and their components.

- Impairments are problems in body function or structure, such as a significant deviation or loss.
- Activity is the execution of a task or action by an individual.
- Participation is involvement in a life situation.
- Activity limitations are difficulties an individual may have in executing activities.
- Participation restrictions are problems an individual may experience in involvement in life situations.
- Environmental factors make up the physical, social, and attitudinal environments in which people live and conduct their lives (World Health Organization, 2001).

The ICF and its language helps professionals define the need for health care and related services, such as the provision of assistive technology. It recognizes that physical, mental, social, economic, or environmental interventions can improve lives and levels of functioning for persons with diseases that affect them at the body, person, and social functioning levels (World Health Organization, 2001). It also characterizes physical, mental, social, economic, or environmental interventions that will improve lives and levels of functioning. Since assistive technology has the potential to improve daily activities and participation in social and physical environments, and thus improve the quality of life of individuals with disabilities, it clearly fits within the ICF. The WHO common health language is used throughout this chapter to discuss the potential impact of appropriate assistive technology.

AT devices, in general, have the potential to compensate for or facilitate immobility; low endurance; difficulty reaching, grasping, or accurately touching keys or switches; and problems with seeing or hearing, verbal communication, and the complex skills necessary for reading, writing and learning. This next section focuses on legislation impacting AT devices and services and specific categories of AT devices as they are related to these areas of human function.

Legislation

Education: The Individuals with Disabilities Education Act (IDEA)

The Individuals with Disabilities Education Act (IDEA), passed in 1997, strengthens academic expectations and accountability for the nation's 5.8 million children with disabilities. One important impact of

IDEA legislation is that it specifies that AT devices and services be provided to children from birth to age 21 to facilitate education in a regular classroom if such devices and services are required as part of the student's special education, related services, or supplementary aids and services (34 C.F.R. 300.308). For students with disabilities, AT supports their acquisition of a free and appropriate public education (FAPE). All Individualized Education Plans (IEPs) developed for children needing special education services must indicate that AT has been considered as a way "to provide meaningful access to the general curriculum" (IDEA, 1997). Further, AT devices and services included as a component of an IEP must be provided at no cost to the student or parents, though the school may use other public and private funding sources that are available.

IDEA (Part C) also includes children before they start school. It covers the needs of children as soon as their developmental differences are noted. It intends that infants and toddlers receive services in the home or in other places, like preschool settings, where possible. The services provided for these children are described in Individualized Family Service Plans (IFSPs). IFSPs include parents, extended family, early childhood interventionists, and other related services personnel in planning, identifying goals, and providing necessary services. IDEA also recognizes that coordination is needed to help families and children with the transition from infant and toddler programs to preschool programs. As a result, students with disabilities are being educated in preschool settings along with typically developing children in an effort to help all children reach the same developmental milestones.

Table 1   Summary of IDEA Assistive Technology Requirements

- AT must be provided by the school district at no cost to the family.
- AT must be determined on a case-by-case basis; if needed to ensure access to free and appropriate public education (FAPE), AT is required.
- If the IEP team determines that AT is needed for home use to ensure FAPE, it must be provided.
- The student's IEP must reflect the nature of the AT and amount of supportive AT services required.
- A parent is accorded an extensive set of procedural safeguards, including the provision of AT to the child.

Source: Office of Special Education and Rehabilitative Services (OSERS).

The American with Disabilities Act (ADA) and the Reauthorization of the Rehabilitation Act (Rehab Act)

The Americans with Disabilities Act (ADA), passed in 1990, clarified the civil rights of persons with disabilities and specified equal access to public places, employment, transportation, and telecommunications. The ADA built on the foundation of the Rehabilitation Act of 1973 (updated in 2003 as the Reauthorization of the Rehabilitation Act) in recognizing the role of employment in enabling individuals with disabilities to become economically self-sufficient and integrated into communities.

Vocational rehabilitation services are often key in enabling employment for adults with disabilities. This legislation mandates AT devices and services be considered and provided as a means to acquire vocational training as well as to enter into and maintain employment. It also requires that AT be considered during the development and implementation of the Individualized Worker Rehabilitation Plan (IWRP), the document that guides a person's vocational rehabilitation process. For example, if an individual is blind and needs to fill out paperwork in order to determine his or her eligibility for vocational rehabilitation services, assistive devices to facilitate reading must be provided at that time. In recent years, Offices of Vocational Rehabilitation have become an important source of funding for AT devices and services to support employment for adults with disabilities.

The Telecommunications Act, Section 255

The Telecommunications Act, first implemented in 1996 and led by the Federal Communications Commission (FCC), requires telecommunications equipment manufacturers and service providers to make their products and services accessible to people with disabilities, as long as this access is readily achievable. These rules are found in Section 255 of the Telecommunications Act. Where access is not readily achievable, these rules require manufacturers and service providers to make their devices and services compatible with peripheral devices and specialized customer-premises equipment typically used by people with disabilities. The FCC has also determined that interconnected Voice over Internet Protocol (VoIP) providers must comply with Section 255.

Products and Services Covered Under Section 255

These requirements cover all hardware and software telephone-network equipment and customer-premises equipment (CPE). According to the FCC,

"CPE is telecommunications equipment used in the home or office (or other premises) to originate, route or terminate telecommunications" (n.d.). This equipment includes telephones, fax machines, answering machines and pagers.

These rules cover basic and special telecommunications services, including regular telephone calls, call waiting, speed dialing, call forwarding, computer-provided directory assistance, call monitoring, caller identification, call tracing, and repeat dialing. In addition, the rules cover interactive voice response (IVR) systems, which are phone systems that provide callers with menus of choices, and voice mail.

Human Technology Interface (HTI)

Considering how each of us interacts with technology gives insight into the issues involved in the concept of Human Technology Interface (HTI). Devices silently wait for activation or input from the people who use them. For example, a stereo or cell phone only responds when a human does something to activate it. A computer only does what it is instructed to do. Even though it may seem like the computer is in charge, the reality is that it only responds to the codes developed and later activated by humans. These activations commonly occur through the use of dials, switches, keyboards, handlebars, joysticks, or handgrips. These interfaces almost always require fine motor control, adequate hearing and/or vision, etc. People know they have successfully interacted with a device by the physical, visual, or auditory feedback these devices provide (e.g., the sight of brewing coffee, images on a computer monitor, or the sound of a phone ringing). Individuals with impairments that affect their interaction with items in their environment may need special consideration in the design, function, or placement of the devices they want or need to activate.

For individuals with complex motor access disabilities, HTI decisions become much more difficult. In these situations, it is critical for clinicians, such as occupational and physical therapists, to consider physical access to technology in a somewhat stepwise progression. This means that it is very important to first consider how the individuals with disabilities are seated or positioned in their wheelchair, bed, or other positioning device.

This essential first step creates the opportunity for individuals to achieve optimal use of any residual abilities they might have, such as reaching with their arm or grasping with their hand. There are any number of orthotic or ergonomic seating and positioning interventions that can be utilized. Once someone is properly seated and/or positioned, the clinician can then move forward with the AT evaluation or intervention. Without this consideration, physical access to ATs and other household technologies can be constrained.

Direct Selection

Once optimal positioning is established, assessment of an individual's reliable, low-effort, high-accuracy hand movements, vision, communication, and hearing will help an evaluator decide whether or not they are able to use a typical "interface" or need one that is adapted. Using a typical interface (e.g., a computer keyboard, steering wheel, TV remote control, etc.) is called "direct selection," since all possible options are presented at once and can be directly selected by the individual. For those without the ability to accurately choose an intended item within the available selection set, a different selection method must be considered.

Scanning or Indirect Selection

Scanning is the most common indirect selection method used by persons with significant motor impairments. A selection set (e.g., a series of pictures or letters) is presented on a display and is sequentially scanned by a light or cursor on the device. The user chooses the desired item by pressing a switch when the indicator reaches the desired location or choice on the display.

Switches come in many styles and are selected based on the body part that will be activating them (e.g., elbow or chin) and the task or setting for using them (e.g., watching TV in bed or using a communication device while eating). A switch can be as simple as a "wobble" switch that is activated by a gross motor movement, such as hitting the switch with the head, hand, arm, leg, or knee. Other switches are activated by tongue touch, by sipping and puffing on a straw, or through very fine movements, such as an eye blink or a single muscle twitch. Regardless, switch use and timing accuracy can be very difficult for new users and must be taught. One common method to teach switch activation and use is to interface a switch with battery-operated toys and games or home/work appliances to increase motivation and teach the concepts used in indirect selection.

Fairly recent developments include eye gaze switches, which calibrate intentional eye movement patterns and select targets, such as individual keys on an onscreen keyboard. Other new developments include brain wave technology (Eye and Muscle Operated Switch or EMOS™) that responds to excitation of alpha waves to trigger a selection. Both of these direct selection methods are undergoing rapid and exciting technical advances, and it is expected that within the next two to five years, many new and exciting applications will be readily available in the commercial market.

Displays

Human technology interface also applies to the process of completing the feedback loop from devices back to the user. Examples include software that enlarges images on a computer display for a person with low vision, flashing alarms for persons without hearing, and devices that convert printed text into synthesized speech or Braille for persons with blindness or learning disability. Recent touch-screen advances and "swipe" technologies are also creating new opportunities for access by persons with a variety of disabilities.

Interestingly enough, for every new technology advance, such as touch screens or the brain control interfaces mentioned earlier, new challenges may also be created for persons with disabilities. Depending on the type and level of disability, previously accessible technologies may actually become less accessible due to these technology advances. A good example of this problem is the cell phone. Many individuals who could use a standard landline touch phone now struggle with the small size and/or touch screens found on recent cell phones. The Telecommunications Act described in this chapter specifically acknowledges issues such as this and phone companies are working to address accessibility issues.

These Human Technology Interface (HTI) concepts apply to all forms of AT, whether they are being used for seating, mobility, communication, using a computer, or control of the basic household appliances found in multiple environments. Good assessment skills and a focus on the client and his or her goals and needs are essential for HTI success and prevention of assistive devices abandonment.

Assistive Technology for Communication Disorders

Vocal communication allows humans to interact, form relationships, and direct the events of their lives to enable choice and participation. Human communication is based on having both receptive and expressive language abilities and the physical capacity to reliably produce intelligible speech sounds. Communication impairment can result from congenital conditions, such as mental retardation, cerebral palsy, developmental verbal apraxia, and developmental language disorders. Other impairments can be acquired through traumatic brain injury (TBI), stroke, multiple sclerosis, amyotrophic lateral sclerosis, tetraplegia, ventilator-dependence, and laryngectomy due to cancer. AT devices that meet the needs of persons with many types of speech and language impairment are commonly called augmentative and alternative communication (AAC) devices, since they can either support or substitute for expressive language impairments. More recently, the term speech generating device (SGD) has entered into the medical vocabulary to differentiate AAC devices from basic computer devices, especially when seeking third-party funding, such as Medicaid and Medicare.

Some individuals are completely unable to speak or have such severe expressive difficulties that they are only able to communicate effectively with those very familiar with them. For these individuals, many devices are available, ranging from simple, low-tech picture books to high-end, sophisticated electronic devices with digitally recorded or synthetic text-to-speech output capable of producing complex language interactions.

While AAC devices are extremely useful to nonspeaking individuals, they do not replace natural communication. AAC device use should be encouraged along with all other available communication modalities, such as gestures, vocalizations, sign language, and eye gaze.

There are no firm cognitive, physical, or developmental prerequisites for using an AAC device. Instead, comprehensive evaluation techniques are used to match the individual's abilities and communication needs with the appropriate AAC technologies. A qualified team of clinicians performs this evaluation with input from the individual and his or her family members, teachers, employers, and others. Since speaking is considered to be a critical human function, many parents and family members wait to seek out AAC devices for children in the hope that natural speech will develop. However, research shows that using an AAC device can actually support verbal language development and can, in fact, increase the potential for natural speech to develop. Children and adults with severe communication impairments can benefit socially, emotionally, academically, and vocationally from using a device that allows them to communicate their thoughts, learn and share ideas, and participate in life activities.

Nonelectronic Systems

Low-tech, nonelectronic AAC systems are often used in addition to an electronic voice output system (or as a backup system in case an electronic device fails or cannot be used during certain activities, such as a swimming lesson). Low-tech systems can be made by using digital photographs, pictures from books or catalogs, or a simple marker to draw letters, words, phrases, or pictures. Picture library software is also available commercially. These software programs (e.g., BoardMaker™ and PCS Symbols™) incorporate thousands of line drawings and pictures that can be used to quickly and easily fabricate a low-tech, nonelectronic communication system.

Adults with progressive diseases such as amyotrophic lateral sclerosis (ALS) or multiple sclerosis (MS) can also choose to use low-tech picture or alphabet boards as a supplement to verbal communication when they experience fatigue during the day, or as their ability to verbally communicate decreases. Many of these adults choose to use both low- and high-tech communication systems depending on the environment they are in and their comfort level with technology.

Electronic Voice Output Systems: Digital Speech

A variation in low-tech communication systems has developed as a result of the manufacture of low-cost microprocessors capable of storing digitized speech. These low-tech, digital voice output devices work like a tape recorder, allowing recording and storing of simple phrases into memory within the device. When the user wants to speak, he or she simply presses a button and the device speaks the prerecorded message.

Devices such as One Step™, Step by Step™, and Big Mac™ are simple and relatively inexpensive, and they are designed to communicate quick, simple messages, such as "Hi," "Let's play," or "Leave me alone." These technologies are often used with very young children who are beginning communicators, or with those who have significant cognitive impairments. They are not appropriate for individuals needing or wanting to communicate complex thoughts and feelings.

Complex digitized devices store several minutes of recorded voice that is usually associated with representative pictures or icons on a keyboard. These devices are often used by people who are not yet literate, have developmental disabilities, or just wish to have a simple device to use when going to the store or out to eat. One example is the ChatBox 40. This AAC device records up to 30 minutes of speech. Digitized (recorded) messages to be spoken are activated by pressing buttons on the keyboard. It also supports numerous switch-scanning options for individuals who are unable to press buttons. The keyboard supports 10 large keys or 40 standard-sized keys. There are 10 levels of messages available, with the ability to move from level to level with up and down arrows. A 2-line, LCD display supports text display of the digitized messages and menu-driven setup utilities.

Electronic Voice Output Systems: Synthetic Speech

Synthesized speech is created by software that uses rules of phonics and pronunciation to translate alphanumeric text into spoken output through speech synthesizer hardware. Voice output systems such as Tango™, VMax™, and EC02™ are examples of high-tech text-to-speech devices with built-in speech synthesis that speak words and phrases that have been typed and/or previously stored in the device. The advantage of these systems is that they allow users to speak on any topic and use any words they wish to use. These systems, which can encode several thousand words, phrases, and sentences, are expensive (costing from $6,000 to $15,000). They form, however, an essential link to the world for people with severe expressive communication disabilities.

All of these voice output systems, whether digital or text-to-speech, can be activated by direct selection (e.g., using a finger or a pointing device such as a mouth stick or head pointer). They can also be activated using indirect selection (e.g., using a scanning strategy or an infrared or wireless switch). In AAC device use an individual will most commonly use a scanning strategy called row-column scanning, in which he or she activates a switch to begin the scan. When the row containing the desired key or icon is highlighted, the user hits the switch again to scan by column; the process is repeated until the desired word or phrase is assembled. While the process can be slow and tedious, indirect selection provides the only means many people have to communicate with others.

Newer AAC devices, such as the DynaVox Maestro™ and the Essence Pro™, come equipped with a camera, Wi-Fi, and Bluetooth capabilities. These devices are lightweight and have speakers, enabling users to be heard in a crowded room. Access to these devices can be achieved through either direct or indirect selection options, and persons using these devices have the ability to say anything they wish to say—just like someone who is able to talk using their own voice.

Among the latest developments for persons who are completely locked in are SGDs that can be activated by a simple eye blink, or by visually gazing or "dwelling" on the desired area of the screen. The DynaVox EyeMax System is one example of this new, advanced access method for communicators who use the DynaVox Vmax. It is comprised of two parts: a DynaVox VMax and a DynaVox EyeMax accessory.

AAC devices differ in mapping and encoding strategies used to represent language, and in storing and retrieving methods used for vocabulary. However, all systems use either orthographic or pictographic symbols, which vary in ease of learning. When selecting a set of symbols for an individual as part of the user interface, it is important to consider these factors and compare them with the individual's cognitive and perceptual abilities. Other key considerations include whether someone is acquiring new language, such as a young child, or if they are an adult with an intact language system who has had a stroke or who may have a degenerative disease such as multiple sclerosis or amyotrophic lateral sclerosis (ALS). These considerations are critical in determining which system is most appropriate for the individual who will be using it.

Portable Amplification Systems

For people who speak quietly due to low breath support or other difficulties with phonation, portable amplification systems are available that function like a sound system in a large lecture hall. The Speech Enhancer™ processes speech sounds for people with dysarthria and enables improved recognition by others. The user wears a headset with a microphone attached to a portable device; the user's clarified voice is projected via speakers attached to the unit. The ADDvox 7 Watt Voice Amplifier Kit™ is another example of a speech amplifier. It uses a microphone headset that is specifically designed for use by persons with speech disabilities. It elevates the vocal volume of people with temporary or permanent voice impairments and can be used by those who rely on an AAC device or voice prosthesis, or who use esophageal speech to communicate with others.

Assistive Technology for Mobility Impairments

Motor impairments greatly affect the ability of individuals to interact with their environment. Infants are compelled to roll, then crawl and toddle to explore their surroundings. Any motor impairment can greatly impact overall development. This is often the situation with cerebral palsy, spina bifida, arthrogryposis, and other diagnoses that impact motor skills. Early intervention and supportive families willing to create modifications and incorporate AT devices into activities can help children achieve developmental milestones.

The loss of acquired motor abilities through trauma or disease is experienced as a severe loss for children and adults and occurs with spinal cord injury (SCI), stroke, multiple sclerosis (MS), amputation, etc. There are many forms of AT that help compensate for impaired motor skills, and they should be introduced as early as possible in rehabilitation to ensure the best possible outcome. For technology purposes, mobility impairments tend to be described in terms of upper- or lower-body impairments. Persons with disabilities may have either or both of these types of mobility impairments.

Upper-Body Mobility Devices

For many individuals with upper extremity difficulties, the need to be independent is paramount. Eating, dressing, bathing, playing, working, and being active in the community can be frustrated without ATs or adaptations to the environment designed to make things accessible. There are literally hundreds of low-tech devices available for persons with fine or gross motor impairment of the upper body. There are devices designed to improve eating, such as scoop plates and utensils with large handles. Adaptations such as poking a pencil through a tennis ball to provide a larger grasping surface for children and adults who are unable to hold a pen or pencil to write is another example of a simple modification. There are orthotics designed to facilitate hand and arm use as well as "arm rests" that are designed to reduce or eliminate arm and/or shoulder weight for those unable to move their arms freely.

These and many other adaptations are limited only by access to materials and/or the imagination needed to figure out how to make things easier for those who struggle with everyday tasks.

Given the importance of computer use in education, training, and employment, many higher-tech AT devices have been developed to give individuals with upper-body mobility impairment, such as poor hand control or paralysis, access to computers. But what if someone is unable to use a standard mouse and keyboard?

Alternate computer keyboards come in many shapes and sizes. There are expanded keyboards such as the Intellikeys™, which provides a larger target or key surrounded by more inactive space than a standard keyboard. Options such as delayed activation response help individuals who have difficulty with pointing accuracy or removing a finger after activating a key. Individuals unfamiliar with a standard QWERTY keyboard layout have the option for alphabetical layout. This is often helpful for young children who are developing literacy skills, as well as for adults with cognitive or visual impairments.

There are also smaller keyboards (e.g., Tash Mini Keyboard™) designed for persons with limited range of motion and endurance. They are also helpful for individuals who type with one hand or use a head pointer or mouth stick to type. These keyboards use a "frequency of occurrence" layout. The home or middle row in the center of the keyboard holds the space bar and the letters in English words that occur most frequently (e.g., *a* and *e*). All other characters, numbers, and functions (including mouse control) fan out from the center of the keyboard based on how frequently they are used in common computer tasks.

Voice recognition (VR) is a mass-market technology that has become essential for computer access for many persons with motor impairment. Instead of writing via the keyboard, VR users write or speak words out loud. The computer processor uses information from the user's individual voice file, compares it with digital models of words and phrases, and produces computer text. If the words are accurate, the user proceeds, if not, the user corrects the words to match what was said. As the process continues, the computer updates its voice file and VR accuracy improves. This software is cognitively demanding yet can offer "hands-free" or greatly reduced keyboarding to many individuals with motor impairment. The most popular voice recognition software today for persons with disabilities is called Dragon Naturally Speaking™. This software can be as accurate as 95%. However, voice training of the software requires roughly a sixth-grade literacy level, and needed corrections for misspellings or word changes can be somewhat cognitively taxing.

Another group of computer input methods includes devices that rely on an on-screen keyboard visible on the computer monitor, such as the Head Mouse Extreme™ and TrackerPro™. The user wears a head-mounted signaling device or a reflective dot on the forehead to select keys on the on-screen keyboard, choose commands from pull-down menus, or direct mouse movement. On-screen keyboards are typically paired with rate-enhancement options like word prediction or abbreviation expansion to increase a user's word-per-minute rate. Word prediction works exactly the same as those autocomplete programs now found on text messaging devices, such as the iPhone or Android phones. Abbreviation expansion allows the user to code certain words or phrases, such as "HRU" for "How are you?" to minimize the need to spend laborious minutes typing each of the letters, spaces, and punctuation. Both word predication and abbreviation expansion for persons with disabilities predate by many years these options that are now readily available and expected by persons without disabilities using currently available text messaging systems.

Today, tablet devices such as the iPad and other similar technologies are creating a new wave of accessibility as well as accessibility issues. An extensive array of inexpensive applications designed by and for persons with disabilities is now available, with many more being uploaded to app stores on a daily basis. In many cases, these applications have been designed by family members or clinicians seeking an accessibility solution or strategy to teach or develop a new skill, to facilitate literacy activities, or to simply provide a game for someone with a disability to play. The caveat "buyer beware" is key in the app world. Many of these tools require purchase before being able to try them out, and in some cases, they provide limited or no value to the customer. In other cases, these solutions can be extremely beneficial. If possible, check with a qualified AT specialist to determine what they may know about the value of a particular application prior to purchase.

Because so many tasks can be accomplished through computers, individuals with disabilities —even those with the most severe motor impairments—can fully participate in life. They can perform education and work-related tasks and monitor and control an unlimited array of devices/appliances at home, work, play, and school.

Lower-Body Mobility Devices

Individuals with spinal cord injury (SCI), spina bifida, cerebral palsy, or other physical disabilities often have lower-body mobility impairments. AT solutions can include crutches, a rolling walker, a powered scooter, or a manual or powered wheelchair. Functional, independent mobility in children and adults with disabilities has been shown to improve cognitive and perceptual skills, reduce learned helplessness, and increase confidence and participation in everyday activities. Provision of the appropriate wheelchair along with proper seating and positioning has a demonstrated impact in the lives of persons with lower-body mobility impairments. Persons who can become independent in their mobility gain or regain access to their local communities, family activities, employment, and/or educational activities.

The decision to go with a manual or powered wheelchair is based on a number of factors, including whether or not the individual has sufficient stamina and strength to propel a manual chair, his or her cognitive and perceptual abilities, as well as safety issues. A qualified physical therapist often works with an occupational therapist, a rehabilitation engineer, and/or the wheelchair vendor in order to assess what type of chair (powered or manual) is best for the individual. Once the initial decision is made as to the type of chair needed, appropriate cushions and other peripherals are determined and fitted precisely to the individual in order to enhance any and all residual skills he or she possesses.

Simple environmental modifications or adaptations, such as installing a ramp instead of stairs, raising the height of a desk, or widening doorways, can be critical facilitators for those who use wheelchairs and might be all that is needed to enhance mobility. For other activities or to increase participation, adding automobile hand controls, adapted saddles for horseback riding, or sit-down forms of downhill skiing and other sports are available.

There are literally thousands of low-tech assistive devices available for persons with motor impairments. Commonly referred to as aids or adaptive devices for completing activities of daily living (ADLs), these devices include aids for personal hygiene, such as bath chairs and long-handled hairbrushes; items for dressing, such as sock aids and one-handed buttoners; adapted toys for play; and many others. Many low-tech mobility aids can be handmade for just a few dollars, while others, such as an adult rolling bath chair, can cost several hundred dollars. All share the common goal of reducing barriers and increasing participation in daily life.

AT for Ergonomics and Prevention of Secondary Injuries

A rapidly growing area of concern for AT practitioners is the development of repetitive strain or stress injuries (RSI) among both able-bodied individuals and individuals with disabilities. While specialized keyboards and mouse control have provided computer access for many individuals, the pervasiveness of computer technology has also increased the possibility of RSI. Over the past few years, an entire industry of AT has developed to deal with repetitive motion disorders.

Computer desks, tables, and chairs used in computer labs, classrooms, and offices do not always match the physical needs of users. When people with and without disabilities spend hours repetitively performing the same motor movement, they can and do develop RSI. Potential solutions include properly supporting seated posture, raising or lowering a chair or desk for optimal fit, implementing routine breaks, and using ergonomically designed keyboards and other assistive technologies. Many of the AT devices described in this chapter (i.e., alternate and specially designed ergonomic keyboards, voice recognition software, and strategies to minimize keystrokes) can also provide useful solutions for individuals with RSI.

Electronic Aids to Daily Living

Electronic aids to daily living (EADLs) provide alternative control of electrical devices within the environment and increase independence in tasks of daily living. This technology is also referred to as environmental control units (ECU). Within the home, EADLs can control audiovisual equipment (i.e., television, video players and recorders, cable, digital satellite systems, stereo), communication equipment (i.e., telephone, intercom, and call bells), doors, electric beds, security equipment, lights, and appliances (i.e., fan, wave machine). EADLs are controlled directly by pressing a button with a finger or pointer or by voice command, or indirectly by scanning and switch activation. Some AAC devices or computer systems also provide EADL control of devices within the environment.

Almost anyone with limited control over his or her environment can benefit from this technology. Children and adults with developmental delays often benefit from low-tech EADLs that increase independence in play through intermittent switch control of battery-operated toys or electrical devices, such as a disco light. For those unable to operate a TV remote control, switches or voice commands to an EADL allow access to devices they would otherwise be unable to control. Many EADLs also accommodate cognitive and visual deficits. For example, an AAC device can display an icon instead of text for a client without literacy or who cannot read English. The same device can also use auditory scanning so that choices can be heard if the client has impaired vision.

EADLs are primarily used in the home, but they can also be used in a work or school setting. An individual can use EADL technology to turn on the lights at a workstation and use the telephone. A child who uses a switch can participate more fully in the classroom by advancing slides for a presentation or by activating a tape player with a story on cassette for the class.

The term EADL was chosen over ECU (environmental control unit) for two primary reasons. First, the term more accurately defined this area of AT by emphasizing the task (i.e., communication is a daily living activity) rather than the item being controlled (i.e., the telephone). Second, the term was chosen to improve reimbursement by third-party providers because the category of ECUs has been poorly funded in the past. In contrast, aids to daily living (ADL) equipment is traditionally funded very well. ADL equipment, which is designed to make the client more independent in a specific daily living task, includes bath seats, toileting aids, built-up spoon handles, and zipper pulls. This equipment is defined by the "daily living" task it "aids."

ECU devices had the same general goal, but the name failed to reflect the goal, particularly to funding agencies. Electronic aids to daily living expand the list of ADL equipment to include equipment that happens to use batteries or plug into the wall, but still shares the same goal– increasing independence in tasks of daily living.

Assistive Technology for Hearing Impairments

Hearing impairment and deafness affect the feedback loop in the human-environment interaction. The inability to hear is commonly recognized as a significant barrier in communication and can compromise safety in situations where sound is used to warn of danger.

Hearing Aids

Individuals who are deaf or hard of hearing deal with two major issues: lack of auditory input and compromised ability to monitor speech output and environmental sound. Assistive technology devices such as hearing aids and FM (frequency modulation or radio wave) systems can be used to facilitate both auditory input and speech output.

Other types of AT devices provide a visual representation of the auditory signal. These include flashing lights as an alternate emergency alarm (e.g., for fire or tornado) or as a substitute for the ring of a phone or doorbell.

Cochlear Implants

When the hearing system is impaired at the level of the middle ear or the cochlea, a highly specialized form of AT is used to create an alternate means of stimulating the auditory nerve. This technology is implanted surgically, with an electrode array placed within or around the cochlear structure. The external portion, a microphone, relays speech and environmental sound to the implanted portion, which is programmed to process and synchronize the sound and stimulate electrodes appropriately. This system requires a battery pack worn on the body or behind the ear (Turkle, 2006). It also requires an experienced audiologist to teach the individual to use the acoustic cues produced by the cochlear implant as a substitute for natural hearing.

TTY/TDDs—"Text Telephones"

Communication for hearing- and speech-impaired persons can be as easy as dialing the phone and typing a text conversation with the use of a teletypewriter (TTY). Also known as a telephone device for the deaf (TDD), a TTY allows a person who does not hear well enough to talk on the phone to communicate his/her message through text. A small device resembling a typewriter couples to the telephone and transmits the text as typed by the user. The person at the other end must have a similar device or use the government-mandated Federal Relay Service provided in each state and territory of the United States. With today's text messaging services available on most cell phones, many individuals who are deaf are choosing to use this more portable service, and TTY's are quickly being replaced by cell phones.

Visual or vibrating systems provide signals to alert individuals about new events and changing circumstances—such as incoming messages and telephone calls, opened doors, fire alarms, and crying babies—and to provide reminders about wake-up and medication schedules. These systems come in many forms, from specially adapted watches to a wide range of switches, lighting systems, and applications that can be used with handheld devices.

Another recent adaptation for persons with significant hearing impairments is computer-assisted real-time translation (CART). This AT solution involves a specially trained typist or stenographer who captures what is being spoken on a computer. The text is then projected onto a display, resulting in close to "real-time" translation. The advantage of this technology is that it can be used by hearing-impaired individuals who are not fluent in sign language as well as others who might need listening help, such as those who use English as a second language. In addition to use in group environments, like conferences or meetings, a variation of this technology can be used to assist a single student or employee in a small setting.

Environmental Adaptations

For individuals who wear hearing aids, there are additional technologies that can facilitate hearing in large rooms or in noisy, crowded environments, such as a restaurant. The Conference Mate™ and Whisper Voice™ are especially designed for these environments. In the case of the Conference Mate™, the person with the hearing loss wears a "neck loop," which acts as an antenna and is capable of broadcasting directly to a hearing aid. A microphone placed near the speaker transmits directly to the neck loop, eliminating background sound. This product is also an excellent solution for office and school environments. The Whisper Voice™ is similar, except it uses a smaller microphone and is more portable. It can be passed from speaker to speaker with sound transmitted to the neck loop and then on to the hearing aid for amplification.

Environmental adaptations can frequently support individuals who are deaf or hard of hearing. For example, a person speaking to someone who has difficulty hearing can take care not to stand in front of a light source (windows, lamps, etc.) and not to overexaggerate or hide lip movements. Gestures can also be helpful.

Assistive Technology for Visual Impairments

The term visual impairment technically encompasses all types of permanent vision loss, including total blindness. Low vision refers to a vision loss that is severe enough to impede performing everyday tasks, but still provides some useable visual information. Low vision cannot be corrected to normal by eyeglasses or contact lenses.

Low-Tech Visual Aids

A variety of AT devices and strategies can help individuals with visual impairments perform daily activities such as reading, writing, personal care, mobility, and recreation. Among low-tech solutions are simple hand-held magnifiers or large print for reading, and mobility devices for safe and efficient travel. High-contrast tape or markers can also be used to indicate hazards, identify what an item is, or show where it is located. There are also simple devices such as individual binocular magnifiers for viewing complex documents or slides for use in schools or business settings.

Other low-tech solutions include using wind chimes to help with direction-finding, using easily legible type fonts such as Verdana (16-point or larger), and using beige-colored paper rather than white to improve the visibility of text. In recreational activities, solutions include beeper balls, three-dimensional puzzles, and outdoor trails with signage called "Braille Trails" designed to improve access to wilderness and other outdoor activities.

Braille text, although less used than in the past due to the advances of computer and other technologies, is still the first choice of many individuals for reading. Many restaurants now provide large-print, Braille, and picture-based menus for customers with a variety of abilities.

Books on tape are another resource for individuals with severe visual impairments. In addition to commercially available tapes for sale and at public libraries, special libraries provide print materials in alternate formats for persons with visual, physical, and learning impairments. Borrowers can arrange to have textbooks and other materials translated into alternate formats. For more information, contact the American Foundation for the Blind or the National Library Service for the Blind and Physically Handicapped (http://www.loc.gov/nls).

With the advent of the Kindle™, Nook™, iPad™, and other tablet devices, the ability to download books, magazines, and newspapers has exploded. Both the general population as well as persons with disabilities can take full advantage of these new and continuously improving technologies. Text-to-speech capabilities as well as print enlargement and enhancement are built in to most of these new technologies. These technologies, and many others under development, are quickly changing the way we view access to text and visual images.

High-Tech Visual Aids

Numerous high-tech solutions exist for persons with visual impairments. Computers outfitted with a speech synthesizer and specialized software such as JAWS™ or WindowEyes™ allow navigation of the desktop, operating system, applications, and documents, as well as the World Wide Web. All text, as well as tags assigned to graphics and computer commands, can be heard by the person using this software. For text that is printed (such as menus, memos, letters, etc.), a technology called optical character recognition (OCR) allows a page scanner and software to convert print documents into digital form. These documents can then be listened to through the computer's speech synthesizer, or converted to Braille or large-print documents that can be printed for later reading.

Another category of high-tech aids are portable note takers with either Braille or speech-synthesizer feedback for the user. These devices are specialized personal digital assistants (PDAs) with calendars, contact lists, and memo and document capabilities, and they can be purchased with either a QWERTY or Braille keyboard. Again, the newer Android and smart phones have many of these capabilities as well and are being rapidly deployed worldwide.

For individuals with some degree of visual ability, screen magnification software such as Zoomtext™ and MAGic™ enable the user to choose the amount (2 times to 20 times) and type of magnification preferred for optimal computer access. Many magnification applications combine enlargement with speech synthesis or text-to-speech for some voice output capability. A recent addition to the list of screen magnification software is Bigshot™. This software is less expensive ($99) and provides fewer features than some other programs. However, it appears to be a highly affordable alternative for users who do not need access to the more sophisticated computer functions. It can also be a good choice for seniors who use the computer for simpler activities, such as e-mail and creating text documents.

Environmental Adaptations

Persons with visual impairments usually keep the setup of their home and work environments constant, since this strategy helps in locating items and with navigation. However, they usually need specialized training for mobility in the community. Individuals with visual impairments can learn to use environmental cues, such as traffic sounds, echoes, or texture of the sidewalk, in combination with mobility aids, like a white cane or a guide dog, for community navigation.

To supplement these less technical aids, some individuals use electronic travel devices that have the capability to detect obstacles missed by a cane, such as overhanging branches or objects that have fallen. This technology (Talking Signs™) utilizes ultrasound or information embedded in the environment expressly for users who have limited vision. Achieving independence in community mobility is hugely demanding for persons with significant visual impairments because of the high cognitive requirements for remembering routes and because environments constantly change. Many individuals use these types of technologies in order to increase their independent mobility in both familiar areas and the larger community.

Newer outdoor navigation technologies are taking full advantage of satellite-based Global Positioning Systems (GPS). GPS technology enables ready navigation and directional cues for persons with visual impairments when combined with voice output systems. Unfortunately, GPS systems are currently unable to provide accurate cues once someone enters a building, but researchers are actively investigating ways to adapt the technology for indoor navigation.

Assistive Technology for Cognitive/Learning Disabilities

Cognitive disabilities include disorders such as traumatic brain injury, intellectual disabilities, developmental disabilities, autism, Alzheimer's disease, learning disabilities, fragile X syndrome, and other disorders, both developmental and acquired. Most individuals in this group have not had the benefit of using AT devices because relatively few products to date have been specifically developed addressing intellectual impairments. In addition, families, teachers, and others providing support services for individuals with cognitive impairments have generally not been aware of AT's usefulness. Most have looked to simple solutions for persons with learning and/or cognitive impairments, using strategies like colored highlighter tape, pencil grips, enlarged text, reminder lists, and calendars. Others try low-tech adaptations like using a copyholder to hold print materials for easy viewing and making cardboard windows to help eyes follow text when reading.

The U.S. Department of Education, National Institute on Disability and Rehabilitation Research (NIDRR), recognizing the need to increase assistive technology development for persons with cognitive disabilities, funded the nation's first Rehabilitation Engineering Research Center for

the Advancement of Cognitive Technologies (RERC-ACT, www.rerc-act
.org) in 2004. This RERC-ACT, recently refunded (2009–2014), is developing a wide range of assistive technologies focused on vocational and literacy skills, service provision, and enhanced caregiving supports for
persons with significant cognitive impairments.

One of the newer developments from the RERC-ACT is the use of intelligent agents to interactively help people with everyday tasks in education, health care, and workforce training. The systems are designed to
assess, instruct, or assist new readers and learners, as well as people who
have speech, language, reading, or cognitive difficulties. The intelligent or
"animated" agent is available on desktop or mobile computing devices. It
is being used to assist persons with cognitive disabilities in learning new
job tasks and/or to prompt persons through various steps within a task.
Other RERC-ACT work includes the development of "batteryless" micro-
power sensors. The elimination of batteries in sensor technologies for persons with cognitive and physical disabilities enables additional prompts
or inputs based on time, weight, location awareness, and other context-
aware sensing capabilities. It enables developers to utilize context-aware
sensors in a multitude of environments and technologies to facilitate the
safety, capacity, and well-being of persons with cognitive disabilities. This
new field of cognitive technologies promises numerous advances during
the coming decades.

Literacy Technologies

There are a number of both low- and high-technology solutions available to assist with literacy development. Individuals who are unable to
read print materials often use books on tape or some of the text-to-speech
software solutions mentioned earlier, such as JAWS™. Co:Writer™ is an
example of a specially designed application that predicts the word or
phrase an individual is trying to spell as he or she begins to type a word.
Other applications (e.g., Write Outloud™ and Kurzweil 3000™) provide
multisensory feedback by both visually highlighting and speaking the
text an individual is generating on the computer.

In addition to those with mobility impairment, voice recognition (VR)
can sometimes be helpful for persons with learning disabilities so significant they are unable to develop writing skills. Voice recognition software
enables such individuals to speak words, phrases, or sentences into a
standard computer word-processing program like Microsoft Word™.

A review or playback feature in the application allows writers to hear the text they have written repeated back to them.

Although VR software is a rapidly developing technology, the reading ability needed to train the software used to generate a voice file hinders its usability by those with significant literacy disabilities. Dragon Naturally Speaking™ has developed a VR version for children aged 9 years and older, but its success rate for children with learning and other cognitive disabilities has not yet been published.

Other limitations of VR include reduced accuracy in the presence of ambient noise (such as that found in a typical classroom), and fluctuating vocal abilities related to fatigue or some types of disabilities. In general, it takes more than 20 hours to train the software to an acceptable level of accuracy (greater than 90%). Although caution is currently in order when prescribing this type of software, the rapid pace of development bodes well for its future use by persons with disabilities.

Other applications for persons with cognitive impairment focus on a range of topics, including academics, money management, personal skills development, behavior training, development of cognitive skills, memory improvement, problem solving, time concepts, safety awareness, speech and language therapy, telephone usage, and recreation and games. These applications come in a variety of options, including training software, manuals, kits, and online curricula.

Prompting Technologies

Recent mainstream technology developments include handheld personal digital assistants (PDAs) and of course the smartphones discussed earlier in the chapter. Assistive technology software developers (AbleLink Technologies, Inc.) have used this technology and developed software applications (PocketCoach™) that provide auditory prompts for individuals with cognitive disabilities. This software can be set up to prompt an individual through each step of a task as simple as mopping a floor, or as complex as solving a math problem. The latest version of this software combines both voice prompts and visual prompts (Visual Assistant™). The individual setting up the system for a user can simply take a digital picture with the accompanying camera and combine the image with digitally recorded voice prompts to further facilitate memory and cognition. One problem that can occur with this type of prompting system lies in how it operates. Essentially, the prompts are provided in a linear or stepwise progression. Should the individual user miss a step or make a mistake, it is often difficult to help the user independently "get back on track" to proceed with the provided instructions. Work is currently underway in a number of laboratories to develop nonlinear or context-aware prompting systems that can recognize when an error has occurred and provide appropriate coaching to assist the end user in correcting the error and then moving forward with the task.

For students with learning/literacy disabilities and/or visual impairments, the Kurzweil™ text reading software or ZoomText™ screen magnification software can facilitate access to written text. The Livescribe™ pen and the EchoPen™ and software can digitally record lectures and, using special paper, can track precisely what handwritten note matches the exact point of the lecture. A lecture or conversation can be uploaded to a computer and then translated from voice to text. For students who struggle with writing and/or hearing, real-time speech-to-text services are also available for a fee to capture lectures or other verbal communications. The notes can be immediately available to the viewer to enhance active participation in lectures, meetings, or other situations.

Accessible Medical Technologies for Practitioners and Patients

Commonly available ATs for use in a medical setting might include height-adjustable exam tables for physicians who use a wheelchair or have short stature. There are visual-readout stethoscopes for medical personnel with less than optimal hearing, as well as electronic amplified stethoscopes. There are digital cuffs for blood-pressure monitoring and FM listening systems to enhance auditory signals. With the advent of the Americans with Disabilities Act, students with disabilities pursuing careers in medicine and other scientific fields are proliferating. This situation has led to an increased awareness of the need to create an accessible medical school environment as well as accessible medical practice sites.

In addition, medical communities are beginning to recognize the critical need to have available instrumentation that enables persons with disabilities to receive medical services. For example, traditional radiology suites require patients to transfer to a specially constructed table for X-rays to be taken, or to stand in front of various X-ray devices for services such as mammography. For many individuals with disabilities, these devices are unusable, painful, and can be very difficult or fatiguing. New designs (mandated via applicable federal regulations, such as the Americans with Disabilities Act) are beginning to take into account these varying patient needs, and these critical technologies are becoming more commonplace in the marketplace.

Selecting Appropriate Assistive Technologies

Abandonment

Practitioners are sometimes surprised to learn that not everyone with a disability enjoys using technology, however useful it might appear. Depending on the type of technology, nonuse or abandonment rates can be as low as 8% or as high as 75%. On average, one-third of more optional assistive technologies are abandoned, most within the first three months (Galvin & Scherer, 1996).

Research has not yet been done to determine the number of individuals who are unhappy with their assistive devices, but who must continue to use them because they do not know about or feel there is another alternative (Galvin & Scherer, 1996). For example, an individual who has just received a new wheelchair that does not meet expectations cannot simply stop using the chair, but must wait until third-party funding becomes available again (typically as long as five years). Alternatively, the individual must engage in potentially difficult and unproductive discussions with the vendor, who has more than likely provided the chair as it was prescribed by the assessment team.

Research does tell us that the main reason individuals with disabilities choose not to use assistive devices is because practitioners failed to consider their opinions and preferences during the process of selecting the device. In other words, the person with a disability was not included as an active member of the team during the evaluation process (Kaye, Yeager, & Reed, 2008; Lepistö & Ovaska, 2004; Scherer, 2004).

Principles of Clinical Assessment

The goal of an AT evaluation is to determine if AT devices and services have the potential to help an individual meet his or her activity or participation objectives at home, school, work, or play. Other goals include: (1) providing a safe and supportive environment for the person with a disability and his or her family to learn about and review available assistive devices; (2) identifying the need for AT services such as training support staff or integrating an AT device into daily activities, (3) performing modifications or customizations needed to make the equipment effective; and (4) and developing a potential list of recommended devices for trial usage before a final selection of technology is made. In addition, the individual and his or her family, as well as the AT team, should specify up front exactly what they hope to achieve as a result of the evaluation (i.e., equipment ideas, potential success with vocational or educational objectives, etc.).

When selecting team members to conduct an AT evaluation, professional disciplines should be chosen based on the identified needs of the person with the disability. For example, if the individual presents with both severe motor and communication impairments, team members should include an occupational or physical therapist with expertise in human-technology interface as well as a speech-language pathologist with a background in working with persons with severe communication impairments and alternative forms of communication (AAC). If a cognitive impairment has been identified, someone versed in learning processes, such as a psychologist, neuropsychologist, teacher, or special educator, would be an appropriate member(s) of the team. If there is an ergonomic issue (i.e., repetitive stress injury), an evaluator with training in ergonomic assessment or a background in physical or occupational therapy is a necessary component for a successful experience.

It is not appropriate for an AT vendor to be called in to perform an AT evaluation. While vendors can and should be members of the evaluation team, it must be recognized that they have a conflict of interest, since they earn a living by selling products. When working with a manufacturer or vendor, it is important to work with a credentialed provider. When requested by the team, vendors demonstrate their products, discuss pertinent features, and assist in setting up the equipment for evaluation and trial usage. However, other team members, including the end user and his or her family, should perform the evaluation and make the final recommendation(s).

Phase I of the Assessment Process

Knowledge within the field of AT continues to expand and change, sometimes on a daily basis, as new technologies and techniques are developed. This knowledge base directly impacts whether the AT device recommended by the assessment team will be used or abandoned by the consumer. As a result of rapidly changing information, the evaluation process continues to be refined. Many researchers are working to develop standardized AT measurement tools (Bodine, 2009), but the fact remains that there are few available resources to guide practitioners who have not received formalized training in AT assessment.

As mentioned earlier in this chapter, the number-one reason AT is abandoned is because the needs and preferences of the consumer are not taken into account during the evaluation process. Other reasons cited for abandonment of devices include:

- changes in consumer functional abilities or activities;
- lack of consumer motivation to use the device or do the task;
- lack of meaningful training on how to use the device;
- ineffective device performance or frequent breakdown of the device;
- environmental obstacles to use, such as narrow doorways;
- lack of access to and information about repair and maintenance;
- lack of sufficient need for the device functions;
- device aesthetics, weight, size, and appearance (Scherer, 1996).

Given the relationship that must develop between individuals and their selected AT devices, it is common sense that these factors be considered during the evaluation process. The AT assessment process has evolved over the past few decades from a random process of trying out any number of devices with the individual, to a team process that begins with the technology out of sight.

Phase I of the assessment process begins when a referral is received. Standard demographic and impairment-related information is collected, usually over the phone. In the majority of cases, cognitive, motor, vision, and other standard clinical assessments have already been performed, and a release of medical information is requested from the individual or his or her caregiver so that information can be forwarded to the team. If appropriate assessments have not been conducted, they are scheduled as a component of Phase II of the assessment process.

Based on the preliminary information, an appropriate team of professionals is assembled and a date is chosen for the evaluation. The team leader takes responsibility for ensuring that the individual with the disability, his or her family, and any other significant individuals are invited to the evaluation.

At the initial meeting, team members spend some time getting to know the individual. Using methods described by Cook and Hussey (2008) and

Galvin and Scherer (1996), the team identifies the life roles of the consumer (e.g., student, brother, musician, etc.) and the specific activities engaged in by the individual to fulfill those life roles. For example, if a young man is a brother, that means he might play hide-and-seek with a sibling, squabble over toys, or otherwise engage in brotherly activities. If he is a musician, then he might want or need to have access to musical instruments, sheet music, or a means to record and/or listen to music.

Next, the team identifies any problems that might occur during the individual's daily activities. For example, the musician might not have enough hand control to manage recording equipment, or he could experience visual or cognitive difficulties with sheet music. It is important to ask specific questions about where and when these difficulties occur (activity limitations). Perhaps problems occur when the individual is tired or not properly positioned, or when he or she is trying to communicate with others. The individual and his or her family members, teachers, peers, or others close to the person with a disability are also asked to describe instances of success with these activities and to discuss what made them successful (prior history with and without technology). By now the team is usually able to recognize patterns of success and failure from the individual's perspective as common limitations across various environments emerge.

Finally, the team prioritizes the order in which to address barriers to participation, and a specific plan of action is developed. This specific plan of action contains "must statements," like "the device must have a visible display in sunlight" or "the technology chosen must weigh less than two pounds or be easily taken from one location to another."

At this point, the team may be reconfigured. For example, if the individual is not properly seated and positioned, he or she is referred to the occupational or physical therapist for a seating and positioning evaluation before proceeding further. Some members of the team may leave after determining that further assessment from their perspective is not needed. In other situations, as additional needs becomes apparent, new members are invited to join the team (e.g., a vision specialist or an audiologist). At all times, the assessment team includes the individual and his or her caregivers as the primary members.

Phase II of the Assistive Technology Assessment

Once the team has agreed upon the specific plan of action and those things that "must" occur, Phase II of the assessment process begins.

The person with the disability and his or her caregivers are asked to preview any number of AT devices that might serve to reduce activity limitations and increase participation in chosen environments. These AT devices are tried along with various adaptations, modifications, and placements to ensure an appropriate match of the technology to the individual.

It is at this point that the clinician's AT skills become even more critical. If trial devices are not properly configured or if the wrong information is given to the consumer, he or she will be unable to make an appropriate selection. Because many devices require extensive training and follow-up, it is essential that realistic information about training and learning time is provided and appropriate resources within the local community are identified. With very few exceptions, the wise course of action involves borrowing or renting the AT device prior to making a final purchase decision. For many individuals, the actual use of technologies on a day-to-day basis raises new issues that must be resolved. For the technology that appears to be best suited for an individual, for instance, local supports or repair options may not be readily available. In these cases, it is best to first identify local resources or local AT professionals willing to seek additional training before sending the device home with the user. Consumers and their families should always be informed so they can make the final decision regarding when and where the equipment will be delivered.

Unexpected benefits of trial use can occur as a result of improved functioning, including changes in role and status. In some cases, these unexpected benefits create an entirely new set of problems. Family partners are often key participants in rehabilitative processes generally, and in AT for persons with complex disabilities in particular. As with any lifestyle change needed to improve health (e.g., diet, exercise), the buy-in and participation of other household members is critical. Interventions designed to engage family in sustained AT use need to move beyond education and the training related to the AT itself, to engage families in proactive lifestyle changes that integrate the AT. Principles and strategies can be adapted from successful approaches to chronic disease management into a more comprehensive approach to helping families integrate AT successfully into daily life. Examples of such strategies include assessing and enhancing family motivational readiness to change, developing behavioral strategies to implement the AT competently, improving self-efficacy for using AT as part of overall lifestyle change, and tracking and providing feedback on implementation success and its link to outcomes.

Often, successful integration of AT into a family for the purpose of helping one person gain independence requires significant role changes within the family. Instead of "doing for" the person with disability, family members are empowering independence with the support of the AT. Family members must identify the meaning and practical impact of such changes on themselves or else old patterns will undermine use of new approaches designed to enhance independence. Professionals tend to focus on the long-term benefits for the person with disabilities, and they must take a broader look at how the AT affects other family members as well. That broader vantage point is a key piece of the assessment of the family's readiness for the changes brought by the AT. It is important to remember that the AT affects more than just the consumer. It also brings about lifestyle change that will impact all members of the family. A key piece of AT assessment and implementation involves engaging close caregivers and family members in conversations about how their behavior will change, or may need to change, as a result of AT acquisition and the potential for increased independence by the consumer.

For most individuals, these problems can be resolved with time, energy, and patience. Others decide that they either prefer the old way of doing things or are interested in adding to or changing the technology once they have had a chance to experiment with it in different settings.

AT professionals, in consultation with team members, should also anticipate future needs (e.g., physical and cognitive maturation or degenerative processes), and final decisions should consider both the expected performance and the durability of the device. Following the trial or series of trials of the various technologies, a formal report should be generated.

Writing the Report

The evaluation report documents the AT assessment process and must include several components. First and foremost, it is helpful to use layman's terms to help case managers, educators, and others unfamiliar with assistive technologies understand the process.

In cases where medical insurance is being used to purchase technology, it is essential to document the medical need for the device(s) within the report. This information will be included in the "letter of medical necessity" required by medical insurers prior to funding approval. For example, the evaluation report might state: "Mr. Jones will use this wheelchair to enable safe and independent mobility in the home and community and to meet the functional or ADL goals as listed." In instances where educational or vocational funding is being requested to purchase the technology, the report should focus on the educational or vocational benefit of the assistive devices and explain how relevant goals will be met with the recommended equipment.

It is also extremely important that all components of the AT device be included in the list of recommended equipment (e.g., cables, ancillary peripherals, and consumable supplies). In many instances, devices are recommended for purchase as a "system." As a result, acquisition can be delayed for months because an item was not included in the initial list. An estimate of the amount of time, cost, and source of training should also be included at this point. Purchasing AT devices without paying for the AT services needed to learn how to use the devices and/or integrate them into identified life activities will result in low use or abandonment (Galvin & Scherer, 1996; Kaye, Yeager, & Reed, 2008; Lepistö & Ovaska, 2004).

Finally, it is also important to include contact information for the vendors who sell the equipment. Many purchasers are unfamiliar with rehabilitation technology supply companies, and acquisition can be delayed if this information is not included in the report.

Physician Responsibilities

Prescribing the Technologies

The American Medical Association recommends the following items be considered when prescribing AT and certifying medical necessity (Schwartzberg, Kakavas, Malkind, Furey, Change, & Chung, 1996).

The physician must provide evidence of individual medical necessity for the specific AT being prescribed and be prepared to talk with insurance company representatives about the medical necessity of complex assistive technologies (e.g., power wheelchairs, AAC devices, etc.). Reviewing a comprehensive assessment report from the AT assessment team should supply all the needed information.

Health insurance requires an "appropriate" prescription that includes mention of the comprehensive assessment process, the individual's motivation, the availability of training, and the potential functional outcome(s) for the patient, as compared to the cost of the products. Success with reimbursement also includes using the appropriate medical necessity forms and prior authorization procedures.

Documentation in the Medical Record

In addition to prescribing and certifying medical necessity on various forms, physicians must maintain complete patient records that include

patient diagnosis or diagnoses;

duration of the patient's condition;

expected clinical course;

prognosis;

nature and extent of functional limitations;

therapeutic interventions and results;

past experience with related items;

consultations and reports from other physicians, an interdisciplinary team, home health agencies, etc.;

a complete listing of all assistive devices the patient is using, including copies of prescriptions and certification forms or letters;

a system to track device performance, including follow-up assessment schedules and lists of professionals and vendors to contact if problems occur.

This comprehensive medical record supplies the background information required to substantiate the need for the AT devices and services, regardless of the funding source.

Funding Letters of Medical Necessity

Physicians are frequently asked to write "letters of medical necessity." Well-written letters of medical necessity help ensure that the AT needs of patients are met. These letters should include the diagnoses (International Classification of Diseases or ICD codes) and the functional limitations of the individual (e.g., balance disorder, developmental delay, etc). In addition, there should be a statement about the patient's inability to perform specific tasks, such as ADLs, work activities, and walking functionally.

For example, individuals with severe communication disorders typically cannot communicate verbally and/or in writing and are often unable to communicate independently over the phone. This functional limitation would also mean they are unable to adequately communicate their health care needs to medical personnel and are therefore unsafe or at risk. These details should be included in a letter of medical necessity.

The letter should also include a paragraph stating why the equipment is necessary. For example, the use of the equipment will allow the patient to

- function independently or improve the patient's functional ability;
- perform independent wheelchair mobility in the home and community;
- return home or move to a less expensive level of care.

The letter should also state whether the equipment will be required as a lifetime medical need, or explain the need if it is of shorter duration.

Next, the letter needs a rationale for choosing this specific equipment. This section requires a description of the specific equipment features and a list of all required components. This list might include

- features that provide safety or safe positioning for an activity;
- cost effectiveness of preventing secondary complications (e.g., pressure ulcers);
- mobility restrictions preventing independent activity;
- access to areas in home, such as bathroom and kitchen;
- durability of the product over its alternatives;
- past experience, interventions, and results (failure of less expensive solutions).

Funding Assistive Technology

The funding sources for AT devices and services fall into several categories. The AT assessment process often helps to identify which source will be used. One source is private or government medical or health insurance. Health insurance defines AT as "medical equipment necessary for treatment of a specific illness or injury," and a physician's prescription is usually required. When writing a prescription for an AT device, it is important that the physician be made aware of the costs and benefits of the devices and be prepared to justify prescriptions to third-party payors. Funding includes not only the initial cost of the device, but the expense involved in equipment maintenance and patient education or training, as well as the potential economic benefits it provides to the patient (e.g., a return to work).

Assistive technology is usually covered under policy provisions for durable medical equipment (DME), orthoses and prostheses, or ADL and mobility aids. With private health insurance, as with government insurance policies, such as Medicaid and Medicare, coverage is based on existing law and regulations. In 2002, AAC devices were included for reimbursement by Medicare. Assistive technology professionals and other health care providers should continually advocate for adequate coverage of AT in all health care plans.

Funding for AT is also available from other federal and state government entities, such as the Veterans Administration, State Vocational Rehabilitation Agencies, State Independent Living Rehabilitation Centers, and State Departments of Education or Social Services. Local school districts might also fund education-related AT for children.

Each agency or program sets criteria for the funding of AT devices based on their mission and the purpose of the technology. For example, vocational rehabilitation agencies pay for AT devices and services that facilitate or help maintain paid employment, and education systems fund AT that enables students to perform or participate in school.

Table 2   Funding Sources for Assistive Technology, Equipment, and Accommodations

Funding Source	Comments	For More Information/Contact
Employer	Required to fund AT only if it meets the criteria for "reasonable accommodation" under ADA	Employer costs can be offset by: ADA Small Business Tax Credit—up to $5,000/ year. Contact IRS via government pages of phone book or http://www.irs.ustreas.gov. WOTC & WtW Tax Credit—up to $2,400/ employee from WOTC and $8,500/employee from WtW. Contact U.S. Dept. of Labor via government pages of phone book or http:// www.doleta.gov/programs/wotcdata.cfm; forms available by calling (877) 828-2050.
Vocational Rehabilitation	One-Stop partner; must qualify for VR services	Contact VR via state One-Stop Center. For more information see http://www.onestops.info/ article.php?article_id=65&subcat_id=503.
Medicare	For people who have Medicare health insurance	Contact local Medicare office via government pages of phone book or CMS at http://www .cms.hhs.gov.
Medicaid	For people who have Medicare health insurance. State may have additional guidelines	Contact local Medicare office via government pages of phone book or CMS at http://www .cms.hhs.gov.
Private Insurance	Varies	Check policy and/or contact carrier.

Funding Source	Comments	For More Information/Contact
Social Security Work Incentives	IRWE—for people on SSI & SSDI PASS—for people on SSI	Contact local Social Security Administration (SSA) office via government pages of phone book or http://www.ssa.gov/work or call (800) 772-1213.
Veterans Affairs	For people who are veterans or dependents of veterans	Contact the VA via government pages of phone book or http://www.va.gov or call (800) 827-1000.
Local Service, Charitable, Religious, and Civic Organizations	Check to see if individual with disability has connection with such an organization	Local community guides and phone books often have listings of such organizations.
Private Foundations	Application procedures and response times vary significantly	Contact The Foundation Center, 79 Fifth Avenue, New York, NY 10003, (212) 620-4230, Fax: (212) 691-1828, E-mail: library@fdncenter .org, Web site: http://fdncenter.org. Each state also has a Foundation Center "cooperating collection."

Funding is generally available for assistive technology, but persistence and advocacy by the AT provider are required for success (Bodine, 2009; Scherer, 1997). The AT provider must also keep abreast of the requirements of various funding sources in order to direct the client to appropriate organizations. Private funding is often available through subsidized loan programs, churches, charitable organizations, and disability-related nonprofit groups. Often, funding from several sources is needed to reduce personal out-of-pocket costs. It is important that the presumed availability of funding not drive the evaluation process and limit the options that are considered for an individual. When the need and justification for a particular AT solution is clear, then it becomes much easier to locate a source of funding and make the case for purchase of the AT device or service.

Beukelman and Mirenda (1998) identify five steps in developing a funding strategy:

- survey the funding resources available to the individual;
- identify funding sources for the various steps in the AT intervention (i.e., assessment, funding, training, etc.);

- prepare a funding plan with the client and family members or advocates;
- assign responsibility to specific individuals for the funding of each step of the AT intervention;
- prepare the necessary written documentation for the funding source so there is a record in the event an appeal is needed.

Conclusion and Future Directions

The world of AT is moving at a very rapid pace, fed in large part by the growth in mainstream technologies and the culture of inclusion that is changing traditional concepts about disability and impairment. Space travel, satellite-supported telecommunications, wireless networks, robotics, new materials with advanced performance properties, miniaturization of integrated circuits, and innovation in batteries and power sources are all crossing over into the field of AT. Federal funding supports Rehabilitation Engineering Research Centers for the development and testing of new assistive technology concepts. Funds also support the transfer of technologies from the federal laboratory system to assistive technology manufacturers. The convergence of these factors is leading to the development of AT products more likely to meet the needs of persons with disabilities.

References

Beukelman, D., & Mirenda, P. (1998). *Augmentative and alternative communication: Management of severe communication disorders in children and adults.* Baltimore, MD: Paul H. Brookes.

Bodine, C. (2009). Assistive technology in physical medicine and rehabilitation. In R. Braddom (Ed.), *Physical medicine and rehabilitation.* Cambridge, MA: Elsevier.

Brown, K. S., DeLeon, P. H., Loftis, C. W., & Scherer, M. J. (2008). Rehabilitation psychology: Realizing the true potential. *Rehabilitation Psychology, 53*(2), 111–121.

Cook, A. M., Polgar, J. M., & Hussey, S. M. (2008). *Assistive technologies: Principles and practice.* St. Louis, MO: Mosby.

Day, H., Jutai, J., & Campbell, K. A. (2002). Development of a scale to measure the psychosocial impact of assistive devices: Lessons learned and the road ahead. *Disability and Rehabilitation, 24*(1–3), 31–37.

Ebner, I. (2004). *Abandonment of assistive technology.* St. John's, MI: Michigan's Assistive Technology Resource. Retrieved from http://www.florida-ese.org/atcomp/_PDF/MATR%20Abandon%200f%20Assistive%20Technology.pdf

Federal Communications Commission. (n.d.). *Guide: Disabled Persons' Telecommunications Act—Section 255.* Retrieved from http://www.fcc.gov/guides/disabled-persons-telecommunications-access-section-255

Galvin, J. C., & Scherer, M. (1996). *Evaluating, selecting, and using appropriate assistive technology.* Gaithersburg, MD: Aspen.

James, P., & Thorpe, N. (1994). *Ancient inventions.* New York, NY: Ballantine Books.

Johnson, A. (2008). *Factors related to the rejection and/or abandonment of AAC devices.* Durham: University of New Hampshire (Department of Communication Sciences and Disorders).

Kawamura, K., & Iskarous, M. (1994). Trends in service robots for the disabled and the elderly. In *Proceedings of the IEEE/RSJ/GI International Conference Intelligent Robots and Systems.* Munich, Germany.

Kaye, H. S., Yeager, P., & Reed, M. (2008). Disparities in usage of assistive technology among people with disabilities. *Assistive Technology, 20*(4), 194–203.

King, T. W. (1999). *Assistive technology: Essential human factors.* Boston, MA: Allyn and Bacon.

Lathan, C. E., & Malley, S. (2001). Development of a new robotic interface for telerehabilitation. In *Proceedings of the 2001 EC/NSF Workshop on Universal Accessibility of Ubiquitous Computing: Providing for the elderly.* Alcacer do Sal, Portugal: ACM.

Lieberman, J., & Breazeal, C. (2007). TIKL: Development of a wearable vibrotactile feedback suit for improved human motor learning. *IEEE Transactions in Robotics,* 919–926.

Lepistö, A., & Ovaska, S. (2004). Usability evaluation involving participants with cognitive disabilities. In *Proceedings of the Third Nordic Conference on Human-Computer Interaction.* Tampere, Finland.

Louise-Bender Pape, T., Kim, J., & Weiner, B. (2002). The shaping of individual meanings assigned to assistive technology: a review of personal factors. *Disability and Rehabilitation, 24*(1- 3), 5–20.

Marchal-Crespo, L., & Reinkensmeyer, D. J. (2008). Effect of robotic guidance on motor learning of a timing task. In *Proceedings of the Second IEEE/RAS-EMBS International Conference on Biomedical Robotics and Biomechatronics.* Scottsdale, AZ: IEEE Societies of Robotics and Automation and Engineering, Medicine, and Biology.

Mataric, M. J., et al. (2007). Socially assistive robotics for post-stroke rehabilitation. *Journal of Neural Engineering and Rehabilitation, 4*(5).

Murphy, E. F., Cook, A. M., & Harvey, R. F. (1982). *Therapeutic medical devices: Application and design* (A. M. Cook & J. G. Webster, Eds.). Englewood Cliffs, NJ: Prentice Hall.

Phillips, B., & Zhao, H. (1993). Predictors of assistive technology abandonment. *Assistive Technology, 5*(1), 36–45.

Reimer-Reiss, M. L., & Wacker, R. R. (1999). *Assistive technology use and abandonment among college students with disabilities.* Greeley: University of Northern Colorado.

Riemer-Reiss, M. L., & Wacker, R. R. (2000). Factors associated with assistive technology discontinuance among individuals with disabilities. *Journal of Rehabilitation, 66*(3), 44–50.

Scherer, M. J. (1993). What we know about women's technology use, avoidance, and abandonment. *Women & Therapy, 14*(3/4), 117–132.

Scherer, M. J. (1997). Assistive technologies: Stuck in a funding quagmire. *Rehabilitation Management, 10*(1), 70–71.

Scherer, M. J., & Wielandt, T. (2004). Reducing AT abandonment: Proposed principles for AT selection and recommendation. Retrieved from http://www.e-bility.com/articles/at_selection.php

Schwartzberg, J. G., Kakavas, V. K., Malkind, S., Furey, P., Change, C., & Chung, M.-S. (Eds.). (1996). *Primary care for persons with disabilities: Access to assistive technology: Guidelines for the use of assistive technology: Evaluation, referral, prescription.* Chicago, IL: American Medical Association.

Technology-Related Assistance for Individuals with Disabilities Act of 1988. Title 29, U.S.C. 2201 et seq: U.S. Statutes at Large, 102, 1044–1065.

Thrun, S. (2002). Probabilistic robotics. *Communications of the ACM, 45*(3), 52–57.

Trease, G. (1985). *Timechanges: The evolution of everyday life.* New York, NY: Warmick Press.

Turkle, S. (2006). *A nascent robotics culture: New complicities for companionship.* AAAI Technical Report Series. Cambridge: Massachusetts Institute of Technology.

Verza, R., Lopes Carvalho, M. L., Battaglia, M. A., & Messmer Uccelli, M. (2006). An interdisciplinary approach to evaluating the need for assistive technology reduces equipment abandonment. *Multiple Sclerosis Journal, 12*(1), 88–93. doi: 10.1191/1352458506ms12330a

Weires, H. (2008). On the front lines: Medical device advancements continue to come from the battlefield. *Medical Device Marketplace Review.* Retrieved from http://www.nerac.com/download.php?id=41

World Health Organizaiton. (2001). *International classification of functioning, disability and health.* Geneva, Switzerland: Author.

Two

Current Issues, Controversies, and Solutions

Even though assistive technology (AT), from very simple to very sophisticated devices, has been around for many years, the actual *field* of assistive technology is still emerging. While substantial progress has also been made in developing thousands of assistive technologies and creating enhanced accessibility for persons with disabilities to mainstream commercial products such as computers and cell phones, funding for these devices and services remains an often-insurmountable barrier.

Persons with disabilities tend to be underserved when it comes to AT not only because they lack awareness of the benefits of AT, but also because the majority of professionals and caregivers associated with them are also unaware of and/or minimally trained in the critically needed evaluations and interventions necessary to support adequate provision of AT devices and services. In too many cases, persons with disabilities are not offered the opportunity to try out AT or accessible mainstream devices because perceptions exist that they will not benefit from the technology or that it is too expensive. This chapter will explore the many problems, controversies, and potential solutions available to the field of assistive technology.

Awareness and Access to Assistive Technology

During the late 1980s, the U.S. Congress formally recognized the growing potential role assistive technologies could play in improving the lives of persons with disabilities. Sponsored by Senators Ted Kennedy (MA) and Tom Harkin (IA), the Technology-Related Assistance for Individuals with Disabilities Act (P.L. 100-407) was signed into law by President Reagan on August 19, 1988. This law provided funding to develop statewide, consumer-responsive information and training programs designed to meet the assistive technology needs of individuals with disabilities of all ages. During the first five years of this legislation, all states and territories received funding specifically designated to "raise awareness and access" to the benefits of AT by and for persons with disabilities. With some variations over the years, this legislation has remained in effect since 1989 and is known today as the Technology Act Program.

But what do *awareness* and *access* to AT mean, and how are these two terms different? Quite simply, AT awareness means knowing ATs exist that might be helpful for specific individuals and situations. Access means knowing where to go for information and acquisition of assistive technology devices and services. It also means being able to get the technology you need, when you need it, and that it is available where you need it (home, school, work, or play).

Awareness

AT can enable individuals with disabilities to live much more independently and, in many cases, to live a completely independent life. But not everyone who could benefit from AT devices and services takes advantage of them. Many individuals do not even know that useful ATs exist for their particular situation. Often caregivers, family members, and professionals are woefully unaware of the myriad devices that are available. So, why don't more people know about AT?

In most cases, AT awareness tends to follow a path of "just-in-time" learning. In other words, unless and until someone has a problem or an identified need, most people do not begin to think about how technology might help their situation. It is a bit like the old conundrum "How do you know what you don't know, if you don't know it?"

For new parents who are just receiving information about their child's disability, there are multiple health care concerns, fear of the unknown, and a period of acceptance in dealing with their child's disability. Thinking about technology applications is not typically on their radar screen in those early stages. Likewise, for children and adults who acquire a disability at a later stage in life, such as a traumatic brain injury, stroke, or other problems, technology may not be the first thing that comes to mind. Few health care providers today are properly trained in AT applications, making it difficult—if not impossible—to share relevant information during hospitalization and early recovery.

What does awareness mean? For many individuals, awareness simply means that some information regarding assistive technology and its benefits for persons with disabilities has been passed on to them, and they know it exists. For others, awareness can range from understanding a specific AT device's purpose and functional application to having full knowledge of AT-related legal requirements. Awareness can also mean integrating technology into the lives and environments of persons with disabilities and demonstrating knowledge of specialty areas of assistive technology (e.g., access, alternative/augmentative communication, computer-based instruction, mobility, positioning, assistive listening and signaling devices, vision technology, environmental control, and activities of daily living). For some individuals, awareness can also mean recognizing the need for ongoing individual professional or educational development and maintaining knowledge of emerging technologies. In later sections of this chapter, educational opportunities designed to build AT knowledge and credentialing programs will be discussed.

Assistive Technology and Access

Even for those who are aware of technology and its potential to help, there are a number of myths surrounding AT devices and services. The first and perhaps most devastating myth is that AT devices and services are tremendously expensive. Among those health care providers, vocational rehabilitation counselors, and educators who do know about technology, many believe that it is cost-prohibitive and are hesitant to mention it to families already overburdened with disability-related expenses.

In some cases, schools and vocational rehabilitation offices are faced with such difficult budget constraints that they avoid bringing up the potential to purchase AT. This situation occurs in large part because they are statutorily responsible for paying for the technologies, and the perception of high cost persists within many of these settings.

In other situations, individuals with disabilities, caregivers, and professionals may think that an AT might be useful, but they may struggle with knowing how to get access to the technology in order to determine if it is the best solution for their particular situation. Although some AT companies are willing to provide short-term leases in order for a potential customer to try out their technology prior to making a purchase decision, the majority are not. While many AT professionals may have a collection of AT in their clinic or school-based program, there are over 30,000 devices on the market today, and chances are the AT professional may not have precisely the equipment needed or the most up-to-date version for a consumer trial.

It is not only potentially difficult to access the myriad technologies that are available, funding streams also have to be identified. Once a device is selected as potentially useful, funding obstacles—such as third-party payor requirements and the associated paperwork—can create enormous frustration, cause delays, and in some cases, stop device acquisition in its tracks. In response to these struggles, there are a number of strategies that can be used to ameliorate funding obstacles. The paragraphs below highlight strategies that can be applied to support access to appropriate AT by consumers, their families, and the professionals providing services.

One key piece of U.S. federal legislation is the Assistive Technology Act of 1998 (AT Act), as amended (P.L. 108-364). This act supports individual states and territories in their efforts to increase the availability of assistive technology by providing financial assistance to implement programs designed to meet the local AT needs of individuals with disabilities. This legislation, mentioned earlier in this and other chapters, supports local efforts to provide information about and access to assistive technology devices and services. Each state is mandated to provide supports to consumers, their families, and professionals in order to increase access to AT devices and services. This goal can be accomplished through a number of state-level activities (RESNA, n.d.).

The state-level activities included within the AT Act Program (ATAP) require state-designated lead agencies to coordinate and collaborate with other state agencies and organizations to provide: (a) assistive technology awareness training; (b) training on the use of technology; and (c) ongoing technical assistance to these agencies and organizations. In order to facilitate device selection and acquisition, each state is also required to provide device demonstrations, financing options, and a program that supports access to equipment. This program could include a loan bank of equipment for trial purposes, funding for consumers to "rent" equipment from manufacturers, or other similar activities. The AT Act Programs have the potential to work with and support individual consumers, their families, and professionals as they work through the myriad problems that arise when AT devices and services are needed and information is sparse.

Accessing Assistive Technology and Early Childhood

Assistive technology devices and services are one of the 17 services required under Part C of the Individuals with Disabilities Education Act (IDEA). According to IDEA, a device is considered a required AT *only* if it relates to the developmental needs of the child. It is *not* required if the device is being provided to meet the medical, daily living, or life-sustaining needs of a child. If the AT device or service is a required early intervention service (regardless of price), it must be included in the "Early Intervention Services and Supports" section of the Individualized Family Services Plan (IFSP).

AT for early childhood refers not just to specific technologies, but also to adapting a child's environment in order to support his/her ability to participate actively in the home, child care program, or other community settings. This participation may include the ability to play successfully with toys and other children, communicate needs and ideas, make choices, and move independently.

For young children, this support often involves low-tech adaptations such as helping a child to sit by building support into a high chair with towels, modifying a spoon by increasing the size of the handle, or making a book easier to look at by putting spacers between the pages. For children with visual impairments, adding texture to an object so they can feel something they cannot see is a great example of a low-tech adaptation. AT for early childhood can also include more sophisticated technology, such as communication or mobility devices.

Unfortunately, many early intervention (EI) service providers have limited knowledge of or experience with AT and its applications for infants and toddlers and, as a result, may not inform families of its potential in promoting and supporting development and learning. Because of this limitation, many EI providers think that AT is too difficult for young children to learn to use or that they need to demonstrate certain prerequisite skills prior to obtaining AT devices or services.

Some providers are convinced that a very young child's use of AT will make things too easy for the child, subsequently discouraging or inhibiting further skills development. Other EI professionals think of AT as primarily high-tech (e.g., computers) and expensive, a view that causes them to wait and make sure a child really needs a particular device before offering to work with the family to obtain the device. As a result of these barriers, roughly 4% of young children with disabilities have AT devices and services identified on their IFSP.

Delaying acquisition of AT devices and services can, and does, inhibit acquisition of developmental milestones by children with disabilities, particularly for those with severe disabilities. Human brains optimize learning during the first two years of life. Providing AT devices and services as early as possible enables children with disabilities (and their families) to take advantage of this window for growth and development.

Process Flowchart

For all children who are being considered for early intervention and/or related services, a general question should be asked: "Could the child benefit from assistive technology to increase access at home, school, and play and within their community?" To respond to this question, a series of four steps guides the decision process. There are slight variations for each age group.

Often referred to as IDEA Part C, or early intervention services, children in this age group receive a screening (Step 1) and, if significant problems are evident, a multidisciplinary evaluation (Step 2). This evaluation should include consideration of the need for assistive technology. It should also include personnel who have training in AT resources, evaluation, and implementation.

If needs are not identified that require special services at the time of the screening or evaluation, the child may be monitored or dismissed.

Table 1   Ages Birth Through 2

Step 1	Step 2	Step 3	Step 4
Screening	Multidisciplinary Evaluation	Eligibility Determination	Development of IFSP

For children with potential problems, consultation and exploration then occurs with the family to determine what resources might be available to the family. These resources include medical benefits such as Medicaid or insurance, Part C or other potential services, community resources for support groups, classes, and preschool or child care options. In Step 3, the multidisciplinary team and family meet to determine if the child is eligible for Part C services as a child with disabilities or developmental delay. If not eligible, the team may decide to monitor development rather than completely dismiss the child. If eligible, the team proceeds with Step 4 of the process, developing the Individual Family Service Plan (IFSP).

If AT has been identified as a necessary service, the appropriate devices and services must then be included within the IFSP. Many EI personnel overlook this step, which has the potential to create additional burdens on the family. Often, EI personnel recommend environmental or other low-tech adaptations without realizing they are actually working with AT. Not including this information on the IFSP as an AT service may prevent families from gaining access to the necessary funding to ensure these adaptations or ATs are provided to their child.

Children who are three to five years of age who are suspected of having a disability are often referred (Step 1) to a local school district multidisciplinary team or a local clinic-based program for screening. Based on those screening results, an evaluation of the child may be conducted to determine if the child may be eligible for special education and related services (Step 2).

Consideration of AT must be part of the multidisciplinary evaluation, including referrals to local AT providers if appropriate. Eligibility determination (Step 3) occurs with the team (including the family) involved in the assessment. For children who are eligible, an Individual Education Plan (IEP) is developed (Step 4). This plan *must* include AT devices and services if they are deemed necessary for the child to have "access to the general education curriculum."

Table 2   Ages 3 to 5

Step 1	*Step 2*	*Step 3*	*Step 4*
Screening	Multidisciplinary Evaluation	Eligibility Determination	Development of IEP

When children are deemed not eligible for special education services, yet have a disability which may interfere with learning or access to the educational environment, they may be eligible for accommodations under Section 504 of the Rehabilitation Act. For example, a child who has a below-elbow amputation may score extremely well on an educational or cognitive battery of tests but still need AT devices, such a one-handed keyboard or voice recognition software, in order to compete successfully in the educational environment. For these children, an IEP is unnecessary as they are able to perform well academically. Instead they receive what is known as a 504 plan. 504 plans are designed to accommodate those school-age children who need accommodations or modifications in order to achieve academic success, but who do not need special education services.

The problem occurs when early intervention personnel and/or schools do not have the requisite resources, including training and equipment, to conduct appropriate evaluations and/or oversee implementation of AT devices and services. In these situations, parents on behalf of their children can be faced with the frustrating task of applying external pressure on the service providers in order to ensure that their children receive the necessary services and benefits they are entitled to have. Often, a call to the State Director of Special Education Services, the District Administrator, or other officials is all it takes to request this service be provided.

If parents are unsuccessful in their request, they can contact their local protection and advocacy center. The AT Act Program described earlier provides funding to the designated Protection and Advocacy (P&A) Program in each state and territory. Called the Protection and Advocacy for Assistive Technology (PAAT) Program, this program was created in 1994 when Congress expanded the Technology-Related Assistance for Individuals with Disabilities Act (Tech Act) to include funding for P&A to assist individuals with disabilities in the acquisition, utilization, or maintenance of assistive technology devices or services through case management, legal representation, and self-advocacy training. These federally funded sites provide technical assistance and information and referral resources to individuals with disabilities and their families regarding AT devices and services. They are also available to help professionals who are in need of advice or support regarding their rights and responsibilities in certain AT-related situations. A listing of PAAT Programs in individual states and territories can be found at http://www.nls.org/paatstat.pdf.

Assistive Technology and Education

In many instances, families only begin to gain awareness of the benefits of AT devices and services when their child is readying to enter school. For children who qualify for special education services, the Individuals with Disabilities Education Act (IDEA) requires that assistive technologies *must be considered* as part of the Individualized Education Program (IEP) process. The IEP process is designed to ensure that children with special education needs are served in their *least restrictive environment (LRE)*. The use of assistive technology devices may facilitate the student's achievement in the LRE.

Process Flowchart

For children without an existing IEP, the 2004 reauthorization of IDEA introduced the Response to Intervention (RTI) method of identifying and providing preliminary support to children with disabilities. RTI incorporates assessment, intervention, and progress monitoring. It uses a multi-tiered, school-wide approach to promote student achievement and prevent behavior problems. "With RTI, schools identify students at risk for poor learning outcomes, monitor student progress, provide evidence-based interventions and adjust the intensity and nature of those interventions depending on a student's responsiveness, and identify students with learning disabilities" (National Center on RTI, n.d.).

Step 1 for this age group without an existing IEP begins at the primary level of RTI and progresses through several identified tiers of intervention. These interventions should also include AT devices or other adaptations when appropriate. *If the devices, adaptations, or interventions are successful, the child may be monitored, but not receive special education services.* If these strategies are not sufficient for the child to receive reasonable benefit from his/her educational program, a formal special education referral

Table 3   Ages 5 to 21

Step 1	Step 2	Step 3	Step 4
RTI Progress Monitoring	Multidisciplinary Evaluation	Eligibility Determination	Development of IEP

is made (Step 2). At this time a multidisciplinary assessment occurs, including consideration of assistive technology and a referral to the local school district or local AT assessment team when appropriate.

Special education eligibility is determined (Step 3) at a meeting of the entire assessment team. The assessment team must include the child when appropriate and his/her parents or legally authorized representative (LAR) as team members. As with the 3- to 5-year-olds, if the child is not eligible for special education and related services, eligibility under 504 should be considered. Should the child be eligible for special education services, an Individualized Education Plan (IEP) is developed (Step 4). It should be noted that, at any time during the RTI process, a parent or public agency may request an initial evaluation to determine eligibility (IDEA, 1990, 2004).

AT must be provided by the school when the IEP team determines that it

- enables the student to perform functions that could be achieved by no other means;
- enables the student to approximate normal fluency, rate, or standards—a level of accomplishment which could not be achieved by any other means;
- provides access for participation in programs or activities which otherwise would be closed to the student on a routine basis;
- enables the student to concentrate on learning, rather than mechanical tasks;
- provides greater access to information;
- supports normal social interactions with peers and adults; or
- supports participation in the least restrictive educational environment.

By providing tools that help a student function more independently and/or more successfully in the regular classroom, assistive technology can impact both curriculum and staff supports that a student requires. Supplementary aids and services include curriculum modifications, support staff, computers and other assistive technology devices, peer support, and speech, occupational, and physical therapies.

The IEP team needs to discuss how the device will be used by the student and how it will be integrated within the regular curriculum. The IEP team should also identify, *in the IEP document*, how the device will be used by the student in the classroom. This information should be shared with the general classroom teachers, who are members of the IEP team, so that they are aware of how it is to be used. Assistive technology should be used to help the student be involved in and progress through the general education curriculum, much as children without IEPs progress.

It is the responsibility of the school district to provide the equipment, services, or programs identified in the IEP. The school district may pay for the equipment, services, or programs itself, utilize other resources to provide and/or pay for them, or cooperatively fund them.

Schools cannot require parents to pay for an assistive technology device or service identified in the student's IEP or require the parents to use their own private health insurance to pay for the device or service. The "free" in "free appropriate public education" is extremely significant regarding students with disabilities who may require assistive technology devices or services. As stated in IDEA and its regulations, all special education and related services identified in the student's IEP must be provided "at no cost to the parent."

Occasionally, schools will ask the parents to access their private insurance to purchase a specific AT device. Medical insurance will only pay for a device if it is deemed "medically necessary." Items such as wheelchairs and augmentative/alternative communication (AAC) devices are most often requested through private insurance because a case can be made that these technologies are medically necessary. For families who are qualified for Medicaid as their primary insurance, Medicaid can often be used to purchase assistive technology devices. However, the parent must give permission for schools to access their private insurance.

There are times when the outright purchase of equipment or devices is not necessary or even advisable. In instances such as these, school districts might consider rental or long-term lease/purchase options. Equipment rentals or long-term lease/purchase options are not intended to be less costly than purchase. However, renting an AT device for a period of time, rather than purchasing the AT, can convey certain advantages that are worth considering, depending on the individual needs of the student. For example, renting equipment might be a reasonable strategy if the child's condition is considered temporary; if the child's condition is expected to improve or deteriorate; or when it is necessary to try out the equipment before purchase for a student. Long-term leasing or lease/purchase agreements also have potential benefits for schools, which include: no obligation on behalf of the school to purchase the device; reduction of obsolete inventory; flexible leasing terms; use of equipment without a lump-sum purchase; upgrading of equipment as improved technology becomes available; and upgrading of equipment as the student's needs change.

Some children with disabilities do not qualify for special education services because their impairment level is such that they can function in the regular education classroom. For example, children with spina bifida may be able to learn just as well as their peers. However, their mobility may be restricted. In these cases, a student may qualify for services through Section 504.

Section 504 of the Rehabilitation Act of 1973 requires public schools to provide students with disabilities with a free appropriate public education and, in addition, ensures that students with disabilities are afforded an equal opportunity to participate in school programs. This means that schools may need to make special arrangements so that students with disabilities have access to the full range of programs and activities offered. For example, a student who needs a wheelchair lift on a school bus to get to school must be provided with this modification. Other modifications which might be required under Section 504 include installing ramps into buildings and modifying bathrooms to provide access for individuals with physical disabilities. Even though required by the law, none of these types of modifications are funded by Section 504. This means that individual schools must provide funding for these accommodations.

Another significant barrier for students involves ownership of a device purchased by a public school. Devices bought by the school belong to the school, not to the student who uses them. When a family moves from one school district to another, the equipment the student has been using does not automatically move to the new school. Assistive technology can go with a student to a new school if the sending school district agrees to sell or give the device to the family or the new school district. Some states have made provisions for students transitioning between schools (such as from middle school to high school) or for those students whose school years are coming to a close. For students who use AT and graduate, or reach the age of 21 and must leave school because they have "aged out," being required to give back their AT to the school can create a very traumatic situation. In some cases, public schools and state vocational rehabilitation (VR) agencies have created agreements enabling VR systems to purchase this "used" equipment from the schools. In other cases, schools may "look the other way" and allow the student to leave school with the AT. Sadly, some school districts do not feel they have the funding or the flexibility to do this, and students are required to give their AT back to the school. This argument is used frequently by schools to encourage parents to purchase their students' AT privately so they are in a position of ownership.

Vocational rehabilitation services, discussed more thoroughly in the next section, are available in every state and territory and are designed to provide vocational supports for working-age adults who seek, or wish to maintain or regain, employment. Although eligibility requirements (set by each state VR agency) must be met by individuals with disabilities in order to receive VR services, this can be a great resource for continuity of support for those who qualify.

Assistive Technology and Employment

For people with disabilities, just like persons without disabilities, obtaining a job is the best route to living as independently as possible. AT can remove barriers to employment and can help workers with disabilities to be more productive. AT devices such as screen readers for people who are blind or who struggle to read written text, magnifiers, and other adapted computer equipment can facilitate job performance. AT devices and services can also provide substantial benefits to employers. For many persons with disabilities, finding employment with a company that is open to accommodating their disability often creates an environment that makes them extremely happy in their job and eager to maintain their employment for as many years as possible.

Finding employment, particularly for persons with disabilities, is much like a job in and of itself. However, state vocational rehabilitation (VR) services help adults and youth with disabilities find and succeed in employment. Many high schools' special education coordinators include VR services in transition planning for students with Individualized Education Plans. The Rehabilitation Act Amendments of 1973 (Rehab Act, as amended) legislated the creation of vocational rehabilitation agencies in every state and territory. Each state was required to establish, within the federal legislation, eligibility criteria for persons with disabilities who live in their state. It is best to check locally to determine what the eligibility criteria are for a particular location.

Local VR counselors work within the community to evaluate their clients' individual needs, make matches with employers, and offer support services for the successful placement of individuals in jobs that fit their skills and abilities. If AT is required for success at a particular job, the device and training may be funded through the VR office. The VR case manager serves as a liaison with the employer to arrange and integrate the AT and employee needs into the workplace.

The services available through each state's vocational rehabilitation system can play a critical role in assisting people with disabilities to enter the workforce. Assistive technology can greatly enhance the employment options for many people with disabilities. Much like the IEP for education, each state VR service is required to create an Individualized Plan for Employment (IPE).

If assistive technology devices and/or services are identified as necessary to achieve employment goals, the IPE must include

- the specific rehabilitation technology services needed;
- how the technology will be provided in the most integrated setting; and
- who will provide the technology and any services related to its acquisition and use (Rehabilitation Act Amendments of 1973).

Assistive technology items and services are available when they are necessary to help someone with a disability become employable. The VR counselor works with the individual to determine whether these items and services are necessary within one of the following categories:

- assessment to determine the technology needed;
- rehabilitation technology services;
- vocational and training services;
- physical and mental restoration services;
- occupational equipment and tools;
- alternative modes of communication;
- transportation services; and
- other goods and devices, including architectural barrier removal.

The Rehab Act defines rehabilitation technology as "the use of technology, engineering, or scientific principles to meet the needs of and address the barriers faced by people with disabilities in areas which include education, rehabilitation, employment, transportation, independent living, and recreation. Rehabilitation technology is divided into three categories: Rehabilitation Engineering, Assistive Technology Devices, and Assistive Technology Services" (29 U.S.C. § 705[30]). State regulations limit rehabilitation engineering services to the time a qualified person spends evaluating the client and designing, fabricating, or modifying assistive devices (9 C.C.R. § 7024.4).

Not only do the statutory requirements often seem complex and difficult to understand for the consumer, but they can also be overwhelming for the vocational rehabilitation counselor charged with implementing them. Many AT devices, such as augmentative/alternative communication (AAC) devices for those who cannot speak, can be very complex.

Unfortunately, very few vocational rehabilitation counselors have received anything but the most rudimentary awareness training in relationship to their role of ensuring that AT devices and services are provided as indicated in the legislation. For many VR counselors who have never worked with these devices, limited access and awareness of the myriad choices and solutions can be overwhelming. Many vocational rehabilitation counselors, just like many educators and health care providers, have not received the training they need to readily identify what AT devices and services might be useful for the individuals they are serving.

Complicating the situation even further is the limitation imposed on state VR systems by the amount of state and federal funding they receive. Because funding can become limited during the fiscal year, states may be required to move to something called "order of selection." Order of selection is implemented when state VR systems are projected to reach the end of their available funding *before the end* of their state fiscal year. When this happens, state VR agencies reduce their services in order to serve those who are most severely impaired. Individuals who are otherwise eligible for VR services, but who do not have a "severe" disability, might find themselves on a very long wait list as funds are simply not available to meet their needs. In such situations, states must wait until the beginning of the next fiscal year to resume services to all eligible clientele.

Americans with Disabilities Act and Assistive Technology

Although IDEA covers AT in the K-12 environment, laws guiding accommodations in the workplace are not as prescriptive. The 1990 Americans with Disabilities Act (ADA) requires employers with 15 or more employees to provide "reasonable accommodations" to help employees who self-identify as having a disability perform the essential functions of their jobs, so long as providing the accommodations does not pose an "undue hardship" to the employer. An undue hardship may relate to the expense or challenges involved with implementing the device into the existing infrastructure at work.

It is the responsibility of the individual to disclose his or her disability to an employer and to request whatever accommodations might be most appropriate. The process of identifying specific accommodations should be negotiated between the employee and the employer. Although someone with a disability might request a high-end solution as their accommodation of choice, employers are not required to provide the exact accommodation requested by the employee. An employee may suggest an accommodation, and the employer may suggest an alternative accommodation, which the employee must consider. The employer has the right to request "medical" documentation and refuse letters from educational specialists. If the employee does not provide such documentation, the employer is not required to provide an accommodation.

One problem faced by employers, and persons with disabilities as well, is the limited understanding surrounding specific tax credits available to businesses that are willing to support the AT devices or modifications needed by their employees with disabilities. The Internal Revenue Code has disability-related provisions of particular interest to businesses as well as people with disabilities. The Disabled Access Tax Credit (Title 26, Internal Revenue Code, Section 44) is available to an "eligible small business" in the amount of 50% of "eligible access expenditures" that exceed $250 but do not exceed $10,250 for a taxable year. A business may take the credit each year that it makes an eligible access expenditure. Eligible small businesses are those businesses with either $1 million or less in gross receipts for the preceding tax year, or 30 or fewer full-time employees during the preceding tax year.

Eligible access expenditures are amounts paid or expenses incurred by an eligible small business for the purpose of enabling the business to comply with the applicable requirements of the Americans with Disabilities Act. These include amounts paid or expenses incurred to remove architectural, communication, physical, or transportation barriers that prevent a business from being accessible to, or usable by, individuals with disabilities, as well as to provide qualified readers, taped texts, and other effective methods of making materials accessible to people with visual impairments. It also includes providing qualified interpreters or other effective methods of making orally delivered materials available to individuals with hearing impairments; acquiring or modifying equipment or devices for individuals with disabilities; or providing other similar services, modifications, materials or equipment (28 C.F.R. 36; 56 C.F.R. 35544).

An example of this type of expenditure might involve XYZ Company, which purchases $8,000 of equipment to meet its reasonable accommodation obligation under the ADA. The amount by which $8,000 exceeds $250 is $7,750. Fifty percent of $7,750 is $3,875. XYZ Company may take a tax credit in the amount of $3,875 on its next tax return. Another example might involve XYZ Company removing a physical barrier in accordance with its reasonable accommodation obligation under the ADA. The barrier removal meets the ADA Accessibility Guidelines. The company spends $12,000 on this modification. The amount by which $12,000 exceeds $250, but not $10,250 is $10,000. Fifty percent of $10,000 is $5,000. XYZ Company is now eligible for a $5,000 tax credit on its next tax return.

There are also tax deductions available when a company removes architectural and transportation barriers for people with disabilities and/or elderly individuals (Title 26, Internal Revenue Code, Section 190). The IRS allows a deduction of up to $15,000 per year for "qualified architectural and transportation barrier removal expenses." Expenditures to make a facility or public transportation vehicle owned or leased in connection with a trade or business more accessible to, and usable by, individuals who are handicapped or elderly are eligible for the deduction. The definition of a "handicapped individual" is similar to the ADA definition of an "individual with a disability." To be eligible for this deduction, modifications must meet the standards established by IRS regulations implementing Section 190.

Most assistive technology accommodations cost very little—usually less than $500—and with the Disabled Tax Credit, the net cost of the assistive technology can be reduced, in most cases, by as much as 50%. Unfortunately, the vast majority of American businesses remain unaware of these tax benefits.

Office of Disability Employment Policy, Job Accommodation Network, and Assistive Technology

The Office of Disability Employment Policy (ODEP) is a sub-cabinet level agency in the Department of Labor. ODEP is charged with "providing national leadership on disability employment policy by building collaborative partnerships and delivering authoritative and credible data to ensure that people with disabilities are fully integrated into the 21st century workforce" (U.S. Department of Labor, n.d.).

ODEP supports the government-funded Job Accommodation Network (JAN). JAN is a free service that offers employers and individuals ideas about effective workplace accommodations. Vocational counselors, employees, or employers can perform individualized searches for workplace accommodations based on a job's functional requirements, the functional limitations of the individual, environmental factors, and other pertinent information. JAN was designed to increase the potential employability of people with disabilities by providing individualized work site accommodation solutions. It offers the following five steps for identifying AT solutions that might be appropriate for a specific job or job task:

define the situation;

explore resources;

choose the AT;

implement AT accommodation(s);

monitor accommodations.

Employers and employees interested in working together to develop individualized solutions can often use the JAN Web site (http://askjan .org) as a tool for finding creative solutions to ensure a safe and effective work environment for the employee with a disability.

In addition to supporting JAN, ODEP also supports a number of other programs, such as the Employer Assistance and Resource Network (EARN). EARN is a resource for employers seeking to recruit, hire, retain, and advance qualified employees with disabilities. EARN supports employers by providing confidential, no-cost consultation and technical assistance, customized training, comprehensive online resources, and links to state and local community-based organizations serving job seekers with disabilities (http://askearn.org/index.cfm).

Both JAN and EARN are good examples of government-supported efforts to facilitate employment of persons with disabilities. Unfortunately, most individuals with disabilities and potential or actual employers remain woefully unaware of the many supports that are available. The unemployment rate for persons with disabilities who wish to work, and absolutely could work, has remained relatively static for many years at roughly 67% to 70%, depending on available statistics. Research has shown that persons with disabilities who do find employment are among the most valuable and loyal members of the workforce. Employers wishing to find dependable workers would do well to seek out employees with disabilities. Often misperceptions regarding the costs of accommodations, or uneasiness regarding what to "do" with an employee with a disability or how to talk with someone who has a disability, constrains employers from employing workers who would be a valuable addition to the team.

Telework and Assistive Technology

Many employers have discovered the benefits of allowing employees to work at home through telework (also known as telecommuting) programs. Telework has allowed employers to attract and retain valuable workers by boosting employee morale and productivity. Technological advancements have also helped increase telework options. President George W. Bush's New Freedom Initiative emphasized the important role telework can have for expanding employment options for persons with disabilities.

In its 1999 Enforcement Guidance on Reasonable Accommodation and Undue Hardship under the Americans with Disabilities Act (revised October 17, 2002), the Equal Employment Opportunity Commission said that allowing an individual with a disability to work at home may be a form of reasonable accommodation. Reasonable accommodation is any change in the work environment or in the way things are customarily done that enables an individual with a disability to apply for a job, perform a job, or gain equal access to the benefits and privileges of a job. The ADA does not require an employer to provide a specific accommodation if it causes undue hardship, i.e., significant difficulty or expense.

Not all persons with disabilities need—or want—to work at home. And not all jobs can be performed at home. But allowing an employee to work at home may be a reasonable accommodation where the person's disability prevents them from successfully performing the job on site, and the job, or parts of the job, can be performed at home without causing significant difficulty or expense.

The ADA does not require an employer to offer a telework program to all employees. However, if an employer does offer telework, it must allow employees with disabilities an equal opportunity to participate in such a program. In addition, the ADA's reasonable accommodation obligation, which includes modifying workplace policies, might require an employer to waive certain eligibility requirements or otherwise modify its telework program for someone with a disability who needs to work at home. For example, an employer may generally require that employees work at least one year before they are eligible to participate in a telework program. If a new employee needs to work at home because of a disability, and the job can be performed at home, then an employer may waive its one-year rule for this individual.

Changing the location where work is performed may fall under the ADA's reasonable accommodation requirement of modifying workplace policies, even if the employer does not allow other employees to telework. However, an employer is not obligated to adopt an employee's preferred or requested accommodation and may instead offer alternate accommodations, as long as they are effective.

The determination of whether or not someone is eligible (as an ADA accommodation) to work from home should be made through a flexible "interactive process" between the employer and the individual. The process begins with an individual first informing the employer that s/he has a medical condition that requires some change in the way a job is performed. The individual does not need to use special words, such as "ADA" or "reasonable accommodation," to make this request, but must let the employer know that a medical condition interferes with his/her ability to do the job.

The employer and the individual should discuss the request so that the employer understands why the disability might necessitate the person working at home. The employee or potential employee must explain what limitations make it difficult to do the job in the workplace, and how the job could still be performed from the employee's home. The employer may request information about the individual's medical condition (including reasonable documentation) if it is unclear whether it is a "disability" as defined by the ADA. The employer and employee may wish to discuss other types of accommodations that would allow the person to remain full-time in the workplace.

In some situations, however, working at home may be the only effective option for an employee with a disability. In order to determine whether or not a job can be successfully performed from home, the employer and employee first need to identify and review all of the essential job functions. The essential functions or duties are those tasks that are fundamental to performing a specific job. An employer does not have to remove any essential job duties to permit an employee to work at home. However, the employer may need to reassign some minor job duties or marginal functions (i.e., those that are not essential to the successful performance of a job) if they cannot be performed outside the workplace and they are the only obstacles to permitting an employee to work at home. If a marginal function needs to be reassigned, an employer may substitute another minor task that the employee with a disability could perform in order to keep employee workloads evenly distributed.

After determining what functions are essential, the employer and the individual with a disability should determine whether some or all of the functions can be performed at home. For some jobs, the essential duties can only be performed in the workplace. For example, food servers, cashiers, and truck drivers cannot perform their essential duties from home. But in many other jobs, some or all of the duties can be performed at home.

Several factors should be considered in determining the feasibility of working at home, including whether the employer will be able to supervise the employee adequately and whether any duties require use of certain equipment or tools that cannot be replicated at home. Other critical considerations include whether face-to-face interaction with outside colleagues, clients, or customers is necessary; and whether the position in question requires the employee to have immediate access to documents or other information located only in the workplace. An employer should not, however, deny a request to work at home as a reasonable accommodation solely because a job requires some contact and coordination with other employees. Frequently, meetings can be conducted effectively by telephone and information can be exchanged quickly through e-mail.

If the employer determines that some job duties must be performed in the workplace, then the employer and employee need to decide whether working part-time at home and part-time in the workplace will meet both of their needs. For example, an employee may need to meet face-to-face with clients as part of a job, but other tasks may involve reviewing documents and writing reports. Clearly, the meetings must be held in the workplace, but the employee may be able to review documents and write reports from home.

An employee may work at home only to the extent that his/her disability necessitates it. For some people, that may mean one day a week, two half-days, or every day for a particular period of time (e.g., for three months while an employee undergoes treatment or recovers from surgery related to a disability). In other instances, the nature of a disability may make it difficult to predict precisely when it will be necessary for an employee to work at home. For example, sometimes the effects of a disability become particularly severe on a periodic but irregular basis. When these flare-ups occur, they sometimes prevent an individual from getting to the workplace. In these instances, an employee might need to work at home on an "as needed" basis, if this can be done without undue hardship.

As part of the interactive process, the employer should discuss with the individual whether the disability necessitates working at home full-time or part-time. (A few individuals may only be able to perform their jobs successfully by working at home full-time.) If the disability necessitates working at home part-time, then the employer and employee should develop a schedule that meets both of their needs. Both the employer and employee should be flexible in working out a schedule so that work is done in a timely way, since an employer does not have to lower production standards for individuals with disabilities who are working at home. The employer and employee also need to discuss how the employee will be supervised.

It should be noted that an employer may select any effective accommodation, even if it is not the one preferred by the employee. Reasonable accommodations include adjustments or changes to the workplace, such as providing devices or modifying equipment, making workplaces accessible (e.g., installing a ramp), restructuring jobs, modifying work schedules and policies, and providing qualified readers or sign-language interpreters. An employer can provide any of these types of reasonable accommodations, or a combination of them, to permit an employee to remain in the workplace. For example, an employee with a disability who needs to use paratransit asks to work at home because the paratransit schedule does not permit the employee to arrive before 10:00 a.m., two hours after the normal starting time. An employer may allow the employee to begin his or her eight-hour shift at 10:00 a.m., rather than granting the request to work at home. Information about these and other types of reasonable accommodations can be found on the EEOC Web site (http://www.eeoc.gov/policy/guidance/html).

Telecommunications Equipment Distribution Programs (TEDP)

For persons who are deaf, hard of hearing (HOH), or have verbal communication problems, gaining access to and using today's specialized telecommunications equipment can be a significant problem. For many citizens, the costs can appear prohibitive and ready information about specific telecommunications devices can be hard to find.

In the United States, 46 states support a Telecommunications Equipment Distribution Program (TEDP) through a monthly surcharge, or tax, on consumer phone services. These funds are designated to be used by consumers with disabilities who struggle with using today's telecommunication equipment because of their disability. The TEDP provides accessible telephone services for individuals who are deaf or deaf-blind, have a severe hearing loss, and/or have a speech impairment.

This goal is accomplished through a combination of both the Telecommunications Relay Services (TRS) and the Telecommunications Equipment Distribution Program (TEDP). Special equipment is available—at no cost—to enhance telephone communication. The equipment includes, at a minimum: amplified telephones, captioned telephones (CapTels), speaker telephones, teletypewriters (TTYs), videophones, and specialized telephone equipment for deaf-blind citizens.

For many consumers, the TEDP promises opportunities for social communication, a way to request emergency help when needed, as well as increased access to employment or educational opportunities. Unfortunately, the TEDP has sometimes been described as a well-kept secret. While this situation is certainly unintentional, learning about this type of program can be problematic for persons with limited electronic communication access. For participating states, outreach and marketing efforts vary, with some states providing a much more intensive marketing program than others. Other potential barriers to accessing this program include the eligibility requirements. Each state determines the level or degree of disability the individual must possess in order to access the program, as well as income levels they must fall into in order to qualify for the free equipment. For persons interested in learning more about the program, a Web site with contact information for the participating states is available (http://www.tedpa.org/StateProgram.aspx).

Assistive Technology and Medical Necessity

As mentioned earlier in this chapter, third-party insurers such as Medicaid, Medicare, and private insurance companies can and do sometimes fund AT devices and services. Some health insurance plans will buy equipment, or pay part of the cost for some assistive technology devices, but it depends on the specific wording of the policy, including the dollar amount available. The devices covered by insurance are typically not listed specifically, but may be included under a generic term like "therapeutic aids." Unless the policy states unequivocally that the equipment is not covered, it makes sense to submit a request for payment to the insurance company, as many will cover *medically necessary* technologies. For third-party insurers, the equipment must be considered medically necessary prior to their approval to fund it. A doctor's prescription and prior authorization from the insurance company are required in order for it to be processed through an insurance carrier.

One of the biggest barriers to convincing medical insurance companies to pay for specific AT devices and services is the lack of clinical evidence-based outcomes research demonstrating the cost benefits of AT as well as the actual patient health benefit of receiving and implementing appropriate AT. Although much more attention is being paid to this issue today, many years of applied clinical research and documentation are needed in order to convince third-party payors that AT devices and services provide a meaningful advantage for their patients.

In almost all cases, medical coverage of AT devices and services has been gained through litigation and significant advocacy efforts by individuals with disabilities, their families, and care providers. As a result, coverage of AT devices is somewhat spotty. For example, Medicare will not pay for a shower seat for a person who is at risk of falling while bathing. However, Medicare will pay for a home health care aide to come to the home and give the patient a bath. This is just one example of the potential cost benefit to our health care system, as well as the potential to enhance privacy and independence for someone with a mobility limitation, by increasing medical coverage of AT devices.

Another barrier concerns the limited knowledge of AT devices and services by the very physicians who are being asked to write a prescription and provide medical justification for a specific device. Physicians, like professionals in education, vocational rehabilitation, and early intervention, are often unaware of the benefits of AT devices and services. Many are uncomfortable prescribing technologies they have never seen or heard about. It often requires a great deal of conversation, documentation, and negotiation in order for a physician to feel comfortable writing a prescription for AT devices and services. Discussed in the previous chapter, the American Medical Association, in coordination with a number of AT specialists, has published guidelines to help physicians understand their rights and responsibilities in relationship to AT devices and services. These guidelines, called *Use of Assistive Technology: Evaluation, Referral, and Prescription,* are "intended to serve as a quick reference and resource, with the goal of clarifying and organizing the evaluation, referral, and prescription process" for physicians (AMA, 1996).

Assistive Technology Assessment

Occupational therapists, physical therapists, and speech-language pathologists are professionals who have training and expertise in clinically recognized areas. All practicing therapists must pass standardized tests and be certified or licensed in their respective fields. However, a therapist may or may not have experience and expertise in assistive technology. This situation creates an enormous barrier for families, particularly those living far from major metropolitan resources, who are trying to identify and locate a knowledgeable professional capable of meeting the AT evaluation and intervention needs of their loved one.

AT specialists have experience and knowledge in AT and may have certification as an Assistive Technology Professional (ATP). It is critically important to determine whether or not these practitioners have expertise or credentialing in assistive technology devices and services prior to engaging them to provide an AT assessment and/or treatment plan. For individuals with disabilities and their families, it is critical to ask questions regarding the breadth and depth of AT experience the clinician might have. How many persons with disabilities have they seen with the same or similar technology requests as the patient in question? What types of AT devices and services have they provided in the past? How many? When and where have they received AT-related training? Do they have the right equipment available to actually do the assessment? Have they written AT assessment reports and "letters of justification" in the past? Were their justifications sufficient to convince a physician and/or third-party payor that the technology was necessary for the individual they were serving?

Rehabilitation engineers are providers who have engineering and/or medical technology backgrounds and may be familiar with AT devices. They may or may not have the clinical experience of working directly with individuals with disabilities and AT devices. Again, it is important to ask about their experience and expertise to determine if they are able to conduct an assessment or make specific recommendations. Rehabilitation engineers may also provide services in nonmedical-related areas such as home modification, work site accommodations, and computer adaptations.

Experienced peer users may be helpful, but their advice almost always reflects personal experience. This personal experience may be very useful when considering durability of a product or actual usage issues. It can often be valuable to speak with someone who has used a similar assistive technology device on a daily basis, as they may have identified both positive and negative aspects of the technology that impact their individual usage. Peer users also provide a contextual perspective regarding their feelings about using a specific technology and the impact this technology may have had on their independence and/or lifestyle.

Many times, AT requires personal fitting, so what is appropriate for one person may not be appropriate for someone else, even if that person has the same disability. Peer users can be good sources of information about vendor services, such as technical support or vendor responsiveness. A successful user may also serve as a cheerleader for the person who has recently acquired new technology and is struggling through the effort of learning to use the device effectively.

Again, the expertise of the clinician is of critical importance, and it is highly recommended that this expertise be determined in advance. Only clinicians with working knowledge of AT devices, applications, and other AT supports can complete a valid AT assessment. Standards for formal AT assessments vary, but a good assessment should verify a need for AT and identify the recommended AT to meet the needs of the consumer. The main goal of an AT evaluation is to determine if AT devices and services have the potential to help an individual meet their activity or participation goals at home, school, work, or play.

Other goals include

1. providing a safe and supportive environment for the person with a disability and his or her family to learn about and test available assistive devices;

2. identifying specific AT services, such as training support staff or integrating an AT device into daily activities, that will support the implementation of new technology;

3. determining whether any modifications or customization are needed to make the equipment work most effectively for the consumer; and

4. developing a list of recommended devices for trial usage before a final selection of technology is made.

When selecting team members to conduct an AT evaluation, professional disciplines should be chosen based on the identified needs of the person with the disability. For example, if the individual presents with both severe mobility *and* communication impairments, team members should include an occupational or physical therapist with expertise in human-technology interface (HTI) as well as a speech-language pathologist with a background in working with persons with severe communication impairments and augmentative/alternative forms of communication (AAC). If a cognitive impairment has been identified, someone versed in learning processes—such as a psychologist, neurolinguist, teacher, or special educator—would be an appropriate member of the team.

An AT assessment often follows the "art" rather than the "science" of assessment. This is true because, as discussed earlier, many AT professionals do not have access to the information they need to become well-trained evaluators. AT researchers are working to develop standardized AT measurement tools, but the fact remains that there are few available resources to guide practitioners who have not received formalized training in AT.

There are a number of steps that must be completed during the AT assessment process. The first step involves identifying the perceived need of the eventual end user. In some cases, participants attending an AT evaluation or referring someone for an AT evaluation may have different perspectives on what the actual need might be. It is critical that this first step be clearly defined and agreed upon by the team. Prior to commencing any evaluation service, the individual and his or her family, as well as the AT team, should specify exactly what they hope to achieve as a result of the evaluation (i.e., equipment ideas, potential success with vocational, recreational, or educational objectives, etc.).

From this list of goals, AT evaluators can then identify specific tasks or activities the persons with a disability either wants or needs to accomplish. For example, the client may need to have more independence in his or her community mobility, but need a wheelchair that is lightweight and easily lifted into the back of a car as the client will not be receiving a wheelchair lift. It is very important to gather background information as well during the initial phase of the assessment. For instance, what are the goals of the individual? Where does he/she live? What is the environment like? Will the technology be used for single or multiple purposes? Does it need to travel with the consumer? What is the individual's longer-term goal? For example, someone may need an adapted computer now to complete educational tasks, with potential new technologies or new adaptations needed later to meet a longer-term goal of entering the workforce.

These initial components should also be supported by standard clinical assessment data, such as physical, sensory, cognitive, and learning abilities, that can be ascertained through the use of available norm-referenced and validated assessment tools. For clients with significant disabilities, some adaptations may need to be made by the clinician in order to achieve this information. For example, if someone is blind, the clinician may need to read the test questions out loud so the individual can provide an answer. In these cases, the adaptations and how the test was administered by the clinician should be documented in the final report.

Once the client and clinical team have determined the level of abilities and goals of the individual, a "feature match" of the equipment can then be completed. Problems often occur during this segment of the evaluation if the clinician has not been properly trained or is not staying abreast of the latest technology innovations. This is often the time that the clinician needs to do his or her homework. Unfortunately, in both schools and clinics, this time is considered "non-reimbursable" and often takes place late at night or when the evaluator can grab a few minutes during a break. Matching an individual's abilities with available equipment features requires a great deal of skill and training. It is critical that this piece of the assessment be done very well.

Once the feature match has been established, the team (including the client) must determine what equipment considerations need to be used to inform the final selection. For example, if a consumer spends a great deal of time outdoors, equipment features such as screen "viewability" in sunlight/darkness and durability in other environmental conditions in which the equipment will be used (cold/heat, rain, snow, etc.) must be taken into account. Transportability, battery life, ruggedness, weight, and size are all critical equipment considerations that must be identified and discussed so a final decision can be made as to the equipment that should be tried out.

Unless there is a truly compelling reason for not completing at least a four- to six-week trial prior to making a final recommendation for purchase, it is almost always in the best interest of the consumer to "try before you buy." As discussed earlier, this trial can be a problem if a ready loan bank of equipment is not available or if the manufacturer does not have a lease policy. If this is the case, it is critical that a return policy be investigated prior to making a purchase. For many consumers and clinicians, equipment that seems to work well in a clinical environment can be an abysmal failure once it begins to be used in real-world situations. In a study done in Colorado by the author's team, over $363,000 were saved by school districts during one school year when students tried equipment prior to making a final purchase recommendation (Melonis, Perkins, Elfner, & Bodine, 2011). Especially when dollars are tight, ensuring that the right equipment is being recommended prior to purchase is a critical component of the selection process for AT devices.

A trial consists of more than providing the equipment to the consumer. This is an area that often breaks down during the assessment process. It is vital that measurable objectives be incorporated within the trial in order to determine if the devices perform well and if the consumer is actually able to use the equipment. The objectives must be reasonable for the available time of the trial, and care must be taken to ensure that the consumer and/or care providers have the available supports they need in order to implement the trial in the environments under consideration (home, school, work, or play).

Once the trial has been completed, it is time to make the final recommendations for all of the components needed by the consumer. Funding sources must be identified and letters of justification written by the clinicians and typically signed by a physician if third-party insurance is being used. If this equipment is being paid for by an educational or vocational rehabilitation system, they will also need to have the proper documentation prior to making the purchase.

One often-forgotten piece of the evaluation process is the training plan. The consumer, caregivers, and clinicians must work together to develop a training plan designed to assist the consumer in learning how to operate the device (device mechanics) and when and how to use it in appropriate situations. For someone who is nonspeaking, for example, the device-appropriate vocabulary will need to be selected and the device programmed or modified for the individual's particular language abilities. Often, the consumer may be a young child or an adult who may or may not be able to learn how to program a sophisticated communication device. In that case, it is imperative that someone within their community be identified to assist with the device. It is equally imperative that a trained AT clinician be available to teach the consumer (and perhaps the caregivers) how to use the device to "talk" with those in their immediate environment. Far too often, technology gets left on the shelf because these steps were not considered during the selection process.

Once the evaluation is complete, the technology has arrived, and training has begun, the team should determine when and how they will reconvene, when to review progress, and what the follow-up plan will be. It is essential that the consumer be an active member of this discussion and be given the opportunity to provide input on when, where, and how these steps would best fit his or her learning and lifestyle.

Credentialing in Assistive Technology Devices and Services

Beyond the standard participation of the various disciplines described in the preceding section, the most widely recognized AT credentialing program is hosted by the Rehabilitation Engineering and Assistive Technology Society of North America (RESNA). RESNA offers national participation for three specialties: (1) assistive technology practitioner (ATP); (2) seating and mobility specialist (SMS); and (3) rehabilitation engineering technologist (RET).

Each credential promotes a standard for recognizing qualifications and validating the broad-based knowledge required as the foundation for safe and effective service in the field of assistive technology. These standards are designed to enhance service provision to people with disabilities who are seeking technology applications to maximize their ability to function.

The RESNA ATP certification program ensures that professionals attain a common level of competence in their ability to provide direct consumer-related services in assistive technology. This program recognizes demonstrated competence in analyzing the needs of consumers with disabilities, assisting in the selection of appropriate assistive technology for consumers' needs, and providing training in the use of the selected devices.

The seating and mobility specialist (SMS) credential is a specialty participation for professionals working in seating and mobility. While the ATP is a broad-based exam covering all major areas of assistive technology, the SMS exam is focused specifically on seating, positioning, and mobility. The program is intended for clinicians, suppliers, engineers, and others involved in seating and mobility service provision. The SMS credential recognizes demonstrated competence in seating and mobility assessment, funding resources, implementation of intervention, and outcome assessment and follow-up.

A rehabilitation engineering technologist is an ATP who applies engineering principles to the design, modification, customization, and/or fabrication of assistive technology for persons with disabilities. The RET certification is active for current certificants but is under review and is not currently available to new applicants.

Problems with AT credentialing to date include the lack of formal recognition by third-party funders such as Medicare and Medicaid, along with the limited awareness, nationally and internationally, that a credential is even available in the field of assistive technology. AT practitioners still have a tremendous amount of work to do to achieve formal recognition of the necessary skills and abilities to conduct safe and effective AT evaluations, implement service plans, and otherwise support persons with disabilities who choose to use AT devices and services.

Navigating Disparities in Assistive Technology Resources

Factors known to be associated with disparities in access to and awareness of AT devices and services include family income, health insurance status, race, and functional ability. Beyond these individual or family determinants, characteristics of the service delivery system, including the quality of service provision, level of public funding, and program eligibility, also contribute to difficulties faced by persons with disabilities and their families.

While it is readily recognized that persons with disabilities have difficulty in basic life activities, the systems that are designed to provide these supports often create untold difficulties for the very individuals they are designed to serve. Having written documentation available in a variety of formats (Braille, large print, audio text) and written in simple language would significantly reduce at least one of the major barriers.

Individuals worldwide are readily able to access the World Wide Web. However, persons with disabilities are the single largest group of individuals without ready access to the Internet. This is true, in part, because so many of them live at or below the federal poverty line. Only 39% of persons with disabilities have Internet access in their own homes. Because of their physical, sensory, or cognitive disability and their need for AT to actually access the computer, those who could benefit the most from ready access to information must often rely on other, able-bodied individuals to provide them with the resource information they need.

For those seeking AT information and supports, navigating the often-overwhelming complexities of the various funding and service systems requires enormous investments of time and energy. The AT Act Program described at the beginning of this chapter is one potential source of information and help for those trying to understand what they need to do in order to access services. RESNA currently serves as a technical assistance center for the Technology Act Programs, and a complete listing of each state's program can be found at http://www.resnaprojects.org/nattap/at/stateprograms.html.

Access to Education About Assistive Technology

There are many educational initiatives on assistive technology being carried out in the United States, Europe, and several other countries. These initiatives are often part of broader programs of physical medicine and rehabilitation, or independent living and self-determination training. However, there has yet to be developed a comprehensive plan of action for ensuring that all relevant disciplinary AT training is provided. For persons with disabilities and their families, the situation is even more difficult, as their access to this information is sporadic at best.

In the United States, minimal preservice education in assistive technology devices and services is being provided to those in special education, clinical disciplines, or engineering, primarily because faculty are undertrained and ill-prepared to teach their students about AT devices and services. Even though the clinical disciplines of occupational and physical therapy and speech-language pathology have adopted standards of practice within their various national credentialing organizations, little formal training is provided to new graduates entering their respective fields.

Assistive technology offers a vehicle to empower people with disabilities to live more independently and participate more fully in their communities. AT service providers are the key professionals needed to assist people with disabilities—and particularly those with significant disabilities—to identify, acquire, and use AT. Without access to qualified professionals and facilities, it becomes difficult, if not impossible, for individuals to be properly evaluated to determine which AT device is most appropriate for them. It may also be difficult for people with disabilities to have AT modified or adapted to fit their individual needs, or to obtain training to use AT more effectively. Advances during the past three decades in both science and engineering have expanded AT options for persons of all ages with disabilities. These advances have led to increased demand for trained service personnel competent not only in the AT devices that are available, but also in assessment and intervention services utilizing assistive technologies.

There is a severe shortage of qualified personnel who have advanced training in the application of assistive technology in the United States, in particular for students with low-incidence disabilities. Jans and Scherer noted in a 2006 publication that the shortage of trained assistive technology personnel creates significant gaps in service delivery nationwide and impairs the acquisition and use of assistive technology (Jans & Scherer, 2006). Additional studies have noted that the lack of trained personnel negatively impacts AT outcomes (Bausch & Hasselbring, 2004; Fitfield & Fitfield, 1997; Mason & Davidson, 2000). The IDEA legislation, Parts B and C, mandates that assistive technology devices and services be provided by early interventionists (for children birth to age three) and educators and allied health providers (kindergarten through twelfth grade) if they are necessary for the child to achieve early developmental milestones or access to the general education curriculum. U.S. educational and early childhood systems are struggling to meet their obligations for assistive technology to be appropriately included in planning and implementing Individual Family Support Plans (IFSPs) and Individualized Education Programs (IEPs) of children with low-incidence disabilities.

Knowledge of policies, research, and best practices in the field of assistive technology is critical to meeting these obligations, and the need for such knowledge continues to increase each year as more children with disabilities enter states' educational systems. While the field of special education has identified clear needs and standards for special educators, it lags in its ability to effectively implement programs that can develop such knowledge and skills (Bausch & Hasselbring, 2004; Laffey, 2004). Although educators often use a range of supplementary aids and services to teach students with disabilities, many educators are not sufficiently familiar with assistive technology to use it effectively. The literature suggests that guidelines and indicators for assistive technology curriculum integration—some broad and some more specific—have advanced significantly (Bausch & Hasselbring, 2004).

Educator competence, however, is lacking when it comes to the specific strategies and applied skills needed to effectively use assistive technology in achieving equal access to the general curriculum for all students with disabilities (Bodine, Donaldson, & Gray, 2001; Gitlow & Stanford, 2003; Laffey, 2004; QIAT Consortium, 2004; SPeNSE, 2002). Even if teachers know what assistive technology is, know what relevant laws and policies are in place, and identify effective models for assistive technology integration, current literature shows that this does not ensure that teachers will be able to identify or use assistive technology effectively to support students with disabilities in their classrooms (COPSSE, 2004; Duffy & Forgan, 2005; Wojcik, Peterson-Karlan, Watts, & Parette, 2004). Definitions, guidelines, laws, and models offer a skeleton for the further development of a true service system (Law, 2008; Lose, 2007; U.S. Department of Education, 2009). Assistive technology can be a powerful tool for educational equity, but only if technology-relevant content and skills are well-learned, well-practiced, and appropriately applied to meet the needs of both the individual and the educational environment (Blair, 2007; Brady, Long, Richards, & Vallin, 2008; NAEP, 2007; Thornton, Peltier, & Medina, 2007; Weintraub & Wilcox, 2006; Wilcox, Guimond, Campbell, & Moore, 2006).

In a study conducted by Long and Perry (2008) regarding pediatric physical therapists' perceptions of their training in assistive technology, the 380 therapists who responded reported receiving less-than-adequate training in AT. They were not confident in their ability to provide AT services, and they indicated weakness in knowledge in the areas of funding technology and services, specific devices, and evaluation methodology. Similar studies across multiple disciplines report much the same. This finding means that new graduates are entering their fields ill prepared to handle the AT needs of their clients.

In the field of speech-language pathology (SLP), the American Speech-Language-Hearing Association (ASHA) published a *Scope of Practice for Speech-Language Pathologists*. This scope of practice defines universally applicable characteristics of practice that speech-language pathologists are responsible for. Because SLPs primarily focus on communication disorders, this document describes the knowledge and practice skills necessary for "establishing augmentative and alternative communication techniques and strategies, including developing, selecting, and prescribing of such systems and devices" for the children and adults they serve.

According to documentation from ASHA,

> AAC is a multidisciplinary field that requires skills that transcend the typical discipline-specific training received by speech-language pathologists, physical therapists, occupational therapists, educators, and other professionals who may serve on an AAC team. Not all SLPs are expected to engage in all areas of AAC practice. However, all SLPs are expected to

recognize situations in which mentoring, consultation, and/or referral to another professional are necessary to provide quality services to individuals who may benefit from AAC.

AAC services should be consumer driven with individuals who use AAC, and their families, playing key roles as members of the team. In most cases the service delivery model of choice is the transdisciplinary approach, encouraging extensive collaboration between team members, role release of skills to and from one another, and maximizing each team member's skills and contributions to the team.

Each team member is expected to possess skills specific to his or her discipline. For example, SLPs are rarely called on to do seating and positioning assessment. Instead, they are more likely to refer to the appropriate team member, often a physical therapist, to carry out such an assessment. These results can have great bearing on the nature of the subsequent AAC device selection and implementation, as do other professionals' findings with respect to individuals' motor skills (and possible means of accessing an AAC device), sensory skills (and implications for size, location, and spacing of items on a communication display), and so on. AAC assessment and intervention requires input from a team, not only an SLP (ASHA, 2002).

However, a survey conducted by Ratcliff, Koul, and Lloyd (2008) of tenure-track faculty and nontenure-track clinical supervisory staff indicated that 29% (49 of 168 respondents) had staff members with AAC as their primary or secondary area of expertise. In contrast, 20% (34 of 168) reported that their teaching staff had minimal expertise in AAC, and another 34% (56 of 168) reported no expertise in AAC within their faculty. Thus, over half of the respondents indicated that their teaching faculty had minimal to no expertise in AAC. Yet graduating practitioners are expected to provide comprehensive AAC services within their sites of practice.

There remains a critical need to develop preservice, in-service, and continuing educational training opportunities in all areas of AT for clinicians and educators working with children and adults with disabilities. The methods used to provide this education can be and are virtually infinite, depending on the amount and extent of the knowledge to be transferred to the end users, the characteristics of the population trained, the environmental context, and so on. With the advent of distance education and high-speed networks, online synchronous and asynchronous coursework is becoming more available and can be accessed 24/7. However, AT training is most effective when trainees have ready access to the equipment they are learning about. In many instances, this component of the training is neglected.

The transmission of knowledge is a process that deals with a somewhat moving target; it never ends because persons change in response to knowledge: new horizons open, new needs arise, and new challenges appear. This means that AT education cannot be solved by providing a simple set of information and notions on a one-time basis. Rather, the field of AT demands ongoing and continuous "just-in-time" training for working practitioners and a solid basis of information at the preservice level.

For individuals with disabilities and their families, training in AT needs to be available in readily accessible formats, and service providers need to know what training exists and how to access this training in order to support their clients. Families often report frustration about their poor access to information, particularly when they need to make an expensive and potentially life-changing decision regarding technology selection.

Technology and Change

In today's world, technology has become ubiquitous. It forms the heart of advanced medical care and daily life for almost all citizens. Yet our use of assistive technology for persons with disabilities lags far behind that of other medical and everyday mainstream technologies. In 2007, the Institute of Medicine's Committee on Disability published its report *The Future of Disability in America*. Key to this report was a series of recommendations related to the $3.9 billion worldwide AT industry. These recommendations included: make needed AT services more available; reduce barriers to health insurance for people with disabilities; and launch a campaign to increase public and professional awareness of assistive and accessible technologies.

Much like commercial, mainstream technologies, AT has undergone constant and rapid change. It is often difficult for AT experts to stay abreast of the latest AT innovations, and with the fairly recent debut of smartphones, tablets, and apps, it is easier than ever to access technology that can make life easier for persons both with and without disabilities. An "app," also known as application software, is defined as computer software designed to help the user to perform singular or multiple related specific tasks. Mobile applications run on handheld devices such as mobile phones (cell phones), personal digital assistants, and enterprise digital assistants.

For funding agencies required to change regulatory or statutory elements in order to fund specific AT devices, keeping up with the rapid pace of technology innovation and change is almost impossible. An example of this problem is the newly developing tablet devices. Many of these tablet devices can be used as AT with the appropriate software or app. Unfortunately, these are considered to be mainstream devices, which are typically unfunded by third-party insurance. Although many payors are working to include these devices within their scope of coverage, as of yet there is no global approach to doing so.

Robotics and robotic systems are also coming to the forefront in the AT field. During the past decade alone, the introduction of robotic technologies into rehabilitation settings has progressed from concept to reality. Numerous studies have demonstrated the efficacy and advantages of rehabilitation robots for assessing and treating motor impairments in both the upper and lower extremities. In addition, numerous university and private industry developers are investigating the efficacy of robotic devices for sensory and cognitive disability applications.

These new developments have been a game changer for many people with disabilities. They are also game changers for professionals working with technology and persons with disabilities. The lines are becoming more and more blurred between specific AT devices and apps that serve a single or a few functions for someone with a disability.

The use of the iPhone, iPod, iPad, and other mobile devices has created a revolutionary new platform for assistive technology. There are now thousands of apps aimed at supporting someone with a disability. In general, they are fairly low in cost. There are also a number of them available that can be downloaded to a mobile device for free. The downside is that most of them have been created by individuals seeking to solve a single "problem," and they have almost all been made available without adequate research to determine their effectiveness for a particular disability. Just because two people have the same diagnosis, it does not mean they will both benefit equally from the same technology.

The other unfortunate side effect of these new apps is the perception by many potential funders that families can be encouraged to purchase the apps and devices themselves, and that will "take care of the problem." This perception, of course, is not necessarily true. What is true is that many of these relatively low-cost apps can be a fabulous solution for specific problem areas and, in some cases, can actually solve what has been a problem for someone with a disability. At the same time, consumers and their families can spend a fair amount of money and end up with a solution that does not work.

Apps are definitely here for the foreseeable future, and they do hold promise for many, many people with disabilities. However, care and concern must still be in place in order to make sure that consumers are not taken advantage of and are not frustrated in their attempts to become as independent as possible.

Conclusion

Assistive technology enables many people with disabilities to live independently, take care of their basic needs, participate in community activities, and engage in gainful employment. But not everyone who could benefit from AT uses it. Some may not know about relevant technologies or appreciate their potential benefits, or may not know how to obtain AT or where to go for good advice; others may need specific devices but not be able to afford them because they are not covered by public programs or private health insurers. Unmet need for AT means that a person is not as fully integrated into society as he or she might be, and may potentially be experiencing social or physical isolation, economic disadvantage, or even failure to meet basic needs. Across disability populations, differences in AT usage may imply that some groups experience relative disadvantage in their ability to be full participants in community life.

Substantial progress has been made in the development of assistive technology devices, including adaptations to existing equipment, that significantly benefit individuals with disabilities of all ages. Such devices can be used to increase the involvement of such individuals in, and reduce expenditures associated with, programs and activities such as early intervention, education, rehabilitation and training, employment, residential living, independent living, recreation, and other aspects of daily living.

Today's technology brings unprecedented opportunity for businesses and workers with and without disabilities. Powerful computers and communications networks have helped create flexible, collaborative, fast-paced workplaces capable of adapting to new markets and labor dynamics. Often, however, companies built these technologies without regard for the needs of workers with disabilities. Adjusting to new technologies is a challenge that all workers face, and for workers with disabilities, it is compounded by the numerous barriers to accessibility they encounter on a daily basis. For example, the Internet is becoming an increasingly visual medium, creating difficulties for those with sensory disabilities. Computer hardware, meanwhile, continues to require levels of fine motor skills that certain individuals with limited mobility or dexterity may not have. The workplace is becoming far more technologically complex, as new software, networks, and applications are accessed from a growing variety of devices, such as computers and mobile devices, requiring workers to constantly adapt to changing technological standards.

Fortunately, innovations in technology represent solutions to the workplace barriers encountered by people with disabilities. E-mail has enabled people with disabilities related to speaking or hearing to be able to communicate effectively and easily, and speech-recognition software has addressed the needs of individuals who have difficulty typing on a keyboard. Frequently, even those without disabilities use these solutions, as when people who are not deaf or hard of hearing use closed-captioning services to improve their comprehension of a video. Many businesses currently implement these technologies in a piecemeal, "add-on" fashion, adopting individual solutions or accommodations for individual workers as needed. A more comprehensive solution requires a broad view of information and communications technology (ICT) infrastructure at the enterprise level, making accessibility requirements not an afterthought or add-on, but an integral design point from the beginning of the process. For the past quarter-century, the accessibility community has advocated for this sort of comprehensive, enterprise-level approach.

References

American Medical Association (AMA). (1996). *Guidelines for the use of assistive technology: Evaluation, referral, prescription.* Chicago, IL: Author. Retrieved from http://www.ama-assn.org/ama1/pub/upload/mm/433/assistivet echnology.pdf

American Speech-Language-Hearing Association (ASHA). (2002). *Augmentative and alternative communication: Knowledge and skills for service delivery.* Retrieved from http://www.asha.org/policy/KS2002-00067.htm

Bausch, M. E., & Hasselbring, T. S. (2004). Assistive technology: Are the necessary skills and knowledge being developed at the preservice and inservice levels? *Teacher Education and Special Education: The Journal of the Teacher Education Division of the Council for Exceptional Children, 27*(2), 97–104.

Blair, M. E. (2007). *U.S. education policy and assistive technology: Administrative implementation.* Logan, UT: Center for Persons with Disabilities, Utah State University.

Bodine, C., Donaldson, C. A., & Gray, K. (2001). *SWAAAC: Supporting learning through assistive technology guidelines,* Version 1.0. Denver: Colorado Department of Education, Special Education Services Unit and University of Colorado Health Sciences Center, Assistive Technology Partners, Department of Rehabilitation Medicine.

Bodine, C., Melonis, M., & Beems, J. (2005). Teaming and assistive technology in educational settings. In D. Edyburn, K. Higgins, & R. Boone (Eds.), *Handbook of special education technology research and practice* (pp. 209-227). Whitefish Bay, WI: Knowledge by Design.

Brady, R. T., Long, T. M., Richards, J., & Vallin, T. (2008). Assistive technology curriculum structure and content in professional preparation service provider training programs. *Journal of Allied Health, 36*(4), 183–192.

Campbell, P., Milbourne, S., & Wilcox, M. (2004). Survey of Part C coordinators and assistive technology. *Research Brief, 1*(4).

COPSSE. (2004). An insufficient supply and a growing demand for qualified related service personnel: Are school districts prepared? *Special Education Workforce Watch.* Retrieved from http://copsse.education.ufl.edu/research-focus-areas/related-services.php?sort=title

Duffy, M. L., & Forgan, J. W. (2005). *Mentoring new special education teachers.* Thousand Oaks, CA: Corwin Press.

Fifield, M. G., & Fifield, M. B. (1997). Education and training of individuals involved in the delivery of assistive technology devices. *Technology and Disability, 6,* 77–88.

Gitlow, L., & Stanford, T. (2003). Assistive technology education needs of allied health professionals in a rural state. *Journal of Allied Health, 32,* 46–51.

Individuals with Disabilities Education Act, 20 U.S.C. 1414(a)(1)(B) (1990).

Individuals with Disabilities Education Improvement Act, 34 C.F.R. § 300.301(b) (2004).

Jans, L. H., & Scherer, M. J. (2006). Assistive technology training: Diverse audiences and multidisciplinary content. *Disability and Rehabilitation: Assistive Technology, 1*(1/2), 69–77.

Laffey, J. (2004). Appropriation mastery and resistance to technology in early childhood preservice teacher education. *Journal of Research on Technology in Education, 36,* 361–382.

Law, W. (2008). What you need to know about IDEA 2004 response to intervention (RTI): New ways to identify specific learning disabilities. *Special Education Law,* 1998–2008. Retrieved from http://www.wrightslaw.com/info/rti.index.htm

Long, T. M., & Perry, D. F. (2008). Pediatric PTs' perceptions of their training in assistive technology. *Physical Therapy, 88*(5), 630–639.

Lose, M. K. (2007). A child's response to intervention requires a responsive teacher of reading. *Reading Teacher, 61*(3), 276–279.

Mason, C., & Davidson, R. (2000). *National plan for training personnel to serve children with blindness and low vision.* Reston, VA: Council for Exceptional Children.

Melonis, M., Perkins, C., Elfner, S., & Bodine, C. (2011). *Annual Report, Assistive Technology SWAAAC Teams.* Denver: Colorado Department of Education.

National Assessment of Educational Progress (NAEP). (2007). *The nation's report card 2007.* Retrieved from http://nationsreportcard.gov

National Center for Response to Intervention. (n.d.). The essential components of RTI. Retrieved from http://www.RTI4success.org

QIAT Consortium. (2004). *Quality indicators for assistive technology services.* Retrieved from http://natri.uky.edu/assoc_projects/qiat/qualityindicators.html

Ratcliff, A., Koul, R. K., & Lloyd, L. L. (2008). Preparation in augmentative and alternative communication: An update for speech-language pathology. *American Journal of Speech-Language Pathology, 17,* 48–59.

Rehabilitation Act Amendments, 29 U.S.C. 722(b)(3)(B)(i)(I) (1973).

Rehabilitation Engineering and Assistive Technology Society of North America (RESNA). (n.d.). Resources for statewide AT programs. Retrieved from http://www.resnaprojects.org/statewide/index.html

Study of Special Needs in Special Education (SPeNSE). (2002). Recruiting and retaining high quality teachers. SPeNSE Summary Sheet.

Technology-Related Assistance for Individuals with Disabilities Act of 1988, Title 29, U.S.C. § 2201 et seq.; U.S. Statutes at Large, 102, 1044–1065.

Thornton, B., Peltier, G., & Medina, R. (2007). Reducing the special education teacher shortage. *Clearing House: A Journal of Educational Strategies, Issues and Ideas, 80*(5), 233–238.

U.S. Department of Education, Office of Special Education Programs. (2009). *Twenty-eighth annual report to Congress on the implementation of the Individuals with Disabilities Education Act.* Washington, DC: Author.

U.S. Department of Labor. (n.d.). ODEP: Office of Disability Employment Policy. Retrieved from http://www.dol.gov/odep

Weintraub, H., & Wilcox, M. J. (2006). Characteristics of early intervention practitioners and their confidence in the use of assistive technology. *Topics in Early Childhood Special Education, 26*(1), 15–23.

Wilcox, M., Guimond, A., Campbell, P., & Moore, H. (2006). Provider perspectives on the use of assistive technology for infants and toddlers with disabilities. *Topics in Early Childhood Special Education, 26*(1), 33–49.

Wojcik, B. W., Peterson-Karlan, G., Watts, E. H., & Parette, P. (2004). Assistive technology outcomes in a teacher education curriculum. *Assistive Technology Outcomes and Benefits, 1*(1), 21–32.

Three

Chronology of Critical Events

Cathy Bodine, Lorrie Harkness, and Maureen Melonis

1808

Pellegrino Turri, an Italian inventor, provides a typewriter to his countess friend who is blind to assist her in writing. He invented it several years prior as others were also working on developing writing machines. The significance of Turri's invention is that it is used as technology for someone with a disability. He is often given credit for inventing the first typewriter. None of these typewriters exist today, but some of the letters the countess typed have been preserved.

1829

Louis Braille, who became blind in his youth, invents a system of raised dots for the blind to use to read. He publishes his work in a book, *The Method of Writing Words, Music, and Plain Song by Means of Dots, for Use by the Blind and Arranged by Them.* The Braille system is still in use around the world today.

1869

Although chairs with wheels for certain individuals with disabilities are mentioned in history as far back as the third century in China, the first patent for a wheelchair is granted in 1869 in the United States. The manual wheelchair has rear push wheels and small front casters. The model is suitable for multiple users.

1876

On February 14 Elisha Gray and Alexander Bell arrive at the patent office in Washington, D.C., within two hours of each other to apply for the first patent for a telephone. Alexander Bell succeeds in being granted the patent to Gray's dismay. The telephone creates a means for remote instantaneous communication. Bell invented his model in the course of trying to develop a hearing aid.

1879

Richard S. Rhodes invents the Audiphone in September. This first hearing aid that works by bone conduction is a device for people who have a specific kind of hearing loss. The device uses a vulcanite fan to transmit air vibrations to the teeth.

1892

On May 27 Frank Haven Hall introduces the Braille typewriter (also called a Braillewriter or Brailler). At the time, he is the superintendent of the Illinois Institution for the Blind. The typewriter types raised Braille dots and is manufactured by the Harrison & Siegfried Company in Chicago, Illinois.

1900

Electrical hearing aids appear. Carbon is used to amplify electrical current. This is the first step away from ear trumpets or conversation tubes. However, these devices are large and awkward to carry.

1916

Harvey Fletcher comes to the Research Division of Bell Labs to work on hearing and speech. He builds the Western Electric Model 2A hearing aid and binaural headset, which is introduced in the 1920s. It uses vacuum tubes to amplify electrical signals, which leads to greater acoustic gain. These early vacuum tubes are very large, with two batteries required for power.

1920

Passage of the Smith-Fess Act (Public Law 66-236) post-World War I brings the expansion of small-scale federal grants for educating veterans and persons with disabilities. The act provides vocational rehabilitation for industrial workers who are disabled on the job.

1927

The first talking film, *The Jazz Singer,* is released in October and becomes a major hit. It is created using a Vitaphone, a sound-on-disc technology. Soon sound on film is the standard for film production, enabling people who are blind to listen to movies.

1931

Congress establishes the Library for the Blind and Physically Handi-capped. A network of libraries begins providing free reading materials to American citizens with visual impairments. Eventually, the service is extended to people with physical disabilities as well.

1932

Harry Jennings, an engineer, builds the first folding wheelchair, the pre-decessor in design to what exists today. It was built for Jennings's friend Herbert Everest, a paraplegic. The Everest & Jennings Company is founded and remains the biggest wheelchair developer for decades.

1934

The Readphone is invented. It reproduces literature and music on discs with over two hours' recording time on each disc. The new tool is useful for the Books for the Blind Project housed within the Library of Congress.

1936

H.W. Dudley, a Bell Labs scientist, invents an artificial talking machine. The world's first electronic speech synthesizer, it requires an operator with a keyboard and foot pedals to supply the pitch, timing, and intensity of speech. Originally called the "voice coder," it becomes known as the "Voder."

1943

The Barden-LaFollette Act, also known as the Vocational Rehabilitation Act (P.L. 78-113), extends vocational rehabilitation services to persons classified as mentally retarded or mentally ill. The new legislation also provides the first federal support for people who are blind and establishes the Office of Vocational Rehabilitation.

1947

During and immediately after World War II, soldiers who become blind in battle are sent to recuperate at Valley Forge Army General Hospital. Richard E. Hoover and C. Warren Bledsoe are assigned to the center to treat the soldiers. A new profession is created called Orientation and Mobility (O&M). Hoover develops a technique for using a long, lightweight cane that revolutionizes independent travel for blind people.

1948

In response to letters requesting textbooks for soldiers who have lost their sight, Anne T. Macdonald of the New York Public Library's Women's Auxiliary launches the Recording for the Blind organization. The GI Bill of Rights provides the soldiers with a college education, but they cannot read the textbooks. Macdonald persuades the women in the auxiliary to read the textbooks aloud and record the words on vinyl phonograph discs to create accessible audiobooks.

1951

David Abraham, a teacher in the Perkins Institute woodworking department, develops the Perkins Brailler. Abraham first presented his Brailler prototype in 1939, but then World War II stopped the production process.

The first Brailler is produced at Howe Press after the war. The same Brailler is used across the world today.

1952

The first speech recognition device (also known as automatic speech recognition or computer speech recognition) converts spoken words to text. Initially the device recognized single spoken digits. Today, speech recognition enables people who are deaf to understand what is being said out loud by reading it as text on a computer screen.

The Tellatouch is developed and provides a means of communication for the deaf-blind person who can read Braille. This unique keyboard provides a method for socialization as well as access to the world for those who are deaf-blind.

1958

On September 2 the Captioned Films Act (P.L. 85-905) is enacted via the Department of Health, Education, and Welfare to provide a loan service of captioned films for persons who are deaf.

The Education of Mentally Retarded Children Act (P.L. 85-926) provides funds to colleges to train teachers to work with students who have cognitive disabilities.

1963

The Mental Retardation Facilities and Community Mental Health Construction Act (P.L. 88-164) provides funds to colleges to train teachers in all disability areas and to conduct research and development on teaching students with disabilities.

1964

James Marsters, a dentist who is deaf, and Robert Weitbrecht, a physicist who is deaf, team up to invent a telecommunications device for the deaf (TDD). A typed conversation is conveyed through a telephone line, opening communication possibilities for the deaf.

1965

P.L. 89-10, the Elementary and Secondary Education Act (ESEA), provides a comprehensive plan for improving the educational opportunities for economically underprivileged children. It provides a statutory basis for the future special education legislation.

P.L. 89-313, the Elementary and Secondary Education Act Amendments, authorizes grants to states to support institutions and state-operated schools in educating students with disabilities. It is the first federal grant program targeting children and youth with disabilities.

1966

The Laser Cane for the blind is introduced. It uses optical triangulation to scan the environment and detect obstacles in the person's path through acoustic feedback. This system becomes a precursor to future attempts to eliminate canes as the primary mode of support for independent travel for people who are blind.

P.L. 89-750, the Elementary and Secondary Education Act Amendments, extends the federal grant program for children and youth with disabilities to the local school level. It also establishes the Bureau of Education of the Handicapped (BEH) and the National Advisory Council (now called the National Council on Disability).

The Education Resources Information Center (ERIC) is established, creating worldwide access to general and special education literature.

The Commission on Accreditation of Rehabilitation Facilities (CARF International) is created through a collaboration between the Association of Rehabilitation Centers (ARC) and the National Association of Sheltered Workshops and Homebound Programs (NASWHP).

1968

P.L. 90-247, the Elementary and Secondary Education Act Amendments, is the last federal special education legislation of the 1960s. It establishes a set of programs that expand and improve special education services nationally and eventually become known as "discretionary programs."

P.L. 90-480, the Architectural Barriers Act (ABA), is enacted. It requires access for people with disabilities to facilities designed, built, altered, or leased with federal funds. Federal agencies are responsible for ensuring compliance with the ABA standards. It is one of the first efforts to ensure access to the built environment.

1970

P.L. 91-230, the Elementary and Secondary Education Act Amendments, which includes Title VI and the Education of the Handicapped Act, establishes a core grant program for local education agencies and eventually becomes known as Part B of the special education legislation.

Closed circuit television (CCTV) is developed to help people with severe visual impairments.

Four members of Stanford University's electrical engineering department, led by Professor John Linvill, develop the technology that becomes the Optacon, one of the first portable electronic print-reading devices. Their incentive is to help John Linvill's daughter, who is blind, to read printed material that has not been transcribed into Braille.

1971

The first two Rehabilitation Engineering Research Centers are funded by the U.S. Department of Health, Education, and Welfare at Rancho Los Amigos Hospital in Downey, California, and Moss Rehabilitation Hospital in Philadelphia. Three additional sites are added in the following year. These centers lay the foundation for research centers on assistive technology for the coming decades.

1972

Arpanet, the U.S. government computer network that was a precursor to the Internet, emerges. Donald Davies of the United Kingdom works on the concept of packet switching, a means by which electronic messages can be broken into tiny "packets" of information in order to travel rapidly from point to point across a network. When scientists and engineers in the United States use the concept of packet switching to develop e-mail applications and Transfer Control Protocol/Internet Protocol (TCP/IP), it marks the beginning of the Internet.

A patent for the first commercial phonetic speech synthesizer is granted to a company that soon becomes Votrax. It is modeled after Richard T. Gagnon's initial work in his basement laboratory, which was motivated by his interest in audio and concern about his own vision loss. This is the beginning of the development of multiple text-to-speech products.

A demonstration of closed captioning is held at Gallaudet College (now Gallaudet University) on February 15. ABC and the National Bureau of Standards demonstrate closed captions embedded within a normal broadcast of *The Mod Squad*. Soon after, open national broadcasts begin on PBS's *The French Chef*, and WGBH follows with several regular broadcast shows having closed captioning. This demonstration initiates a drive, later enacted through legislation, to ensure that television shows are accessible to people with hearing impairments.

1973

The Rehabilitation Act (P.L. 93-112) makes it illegal for organizations to discriminate against people with disabilities and mandates greater equality in the workplace. Sections 501 and 504 of the act require agencies to prevent workplace discrimination as well as to provide accommodations for employees to do their work and for members of the public with disabilities to have access to the agency. In addition, the Rehabilitation Act identifies rehabilitation engineering as a priority of the research and development programs of Rehabilitation Services under the Department of Health, Education, and Welfare. The priorities and requirements of this act become fundamental to the requirements for Rehabilitation Engineering Research Centers (RERCs) of the future.

1974

P.L. 93-280, the Education Amendments, adds to two existing laws: the Education of the Handicapped Act, which for the first time mentions "an appropriate education" for all children with disabilities; and the Family Education Rights and Privacy Act, which gives parents and students over the age of 18 the right to examine educational records kept in the student's personal file.

1975

In July, Massachusetts-based Duxbury Systems introduces the Duxbury Braille Translator, which is the first commercial Braille translator for computers. It allows translation from text to Braille and Braille to text on a computer.

P.L. 94-142, the Education for All Handicapped Children Act (EAHCA), mandates a free appropriate public education (FAPE) for all children with disabilities. The legislation ensures due process rights, requires the preparation of Individualized Education Plans (IEPs), and mandates that education be provided in the Least Restrictive Environment (LRE). It takes effect in October of 1977.

Ray Kurzweil and his team at Kurzweil Computer Products develop the Kurzweil Reading Machine and the first omni-font optical character recognition (OCR) technology, which gives people who are blind access to printed materials. Libraries and schools begin using these machines in the near future.

Bill Gates and Paul Allen establish Microsoft.

1976

Telesensory Systems introduces the first commercial speaking electronic calculator, Speech +. This is a very early use of speech synthesis in a consumer product. The device is quickly sought after by people who are blind.

1977

On April 16 the first pre-assembled personal computer, Apple II, is introduced at the first West Coast Computer Faire. It comes with color graphics and a 5 ¼ inch floppy disk drive and interface.

1978

The National Institute of Handicapped Research (NIHR) is established.

Dean Blazie introduces TotalTalk, the first full-speech talking terminal that can speak for those who cannot speak for themselves. Evolving from earlier speech synthesis technology, it launches the development of new and improved augmentative/alternative communication (AAC) products.

RESNA (Rehabilitation Engineering and Assistive Technology Society of North America) is created as a new organization dedicated to improving the quality of life of persons with disabilities. Assistive Technology becomes recognized as a new area of rehabilitation engineering.

1979

Telesensory Systems introduces VersaBraille, a personal computer for the blind that has a refreshable Braille display system. It opens doors for the blind to work on an equal basis with others on computers.

1981

The IBM Personal Computer is introduced on August 12. The term "personal computer" was used as early as 1972 to characterize Xerox PARC's Alto, but because of the success of the IBM Personal Computer, the term "PC" comes to mean technology that is compatible with IBM's PC products.

1982

G. K. Poock conducts a study that compares the speed and accuracy of speech input versus typed input on computers using a 180-word vocabulary. After he achieves 96.8% recognition accuracy, speech recognition becomes a valid option for computer input.

The U.S. Office of Technology Assessment (OTA) issues "Technology and Handicapped People," a primary federal examination of the impact of technology for people with disabilities. This report emphasizes the need to develop policies aimed at increasing research on technology for people with disabilities, reducing financial barriers to the use of such technologies, and training personnel in disability-related disciplines and services.

1983

Budd and Dolores Hagen establish Closing The Gap as a result of their personal experiences raising a child who is deaf. The organization focuses on assistive technology for people with special needs through a magazine, an annual international conference, and extensive resources on its Web site.

INFO, the first talking database program, is announced at Computer Aids of Ft. Wayne, Indiana. It works with the Echo II voice synthesizer.

In July the Teachers College of Columbia University holds its first summer institute program, "Technology in the Education and Rehabilitation of the Visually Impaired." The program, organized by Larry Gardner and Frank Irzyk, emphasizes practical applications in the use of technology and includes hands-on experience with a variety of assistive technologies.

Time magazine names the computer as its "Man of the Year" for 1982.

1984

Apple introduces the Macintosh computer.

The musical keyboard with acoustic sound is introduced, expanding the world of musical performance and recording for people with disabilities.

Computer Conversations releases the Enhanced PC Talking Program, a DOS screen reader written by Ronald Hutchinson. It works with most of the software written for the IBM PC with the exception of graphics.

1985

AbleData is established to provide a searchable database of objective information on assistive technology and rehabilitation equipment to consumers, organizations, professionals, and caregivers.

Dr. Gregg Vanderheiden and the Trace Center of the University of Wisconsin-Madison work with the computer industry to incorporate accessibility features.

1986

The Rehabilitation Act Amendments (P.L. 99-457) requires states to include a provision for assistive technology services in the Individualized Written Rehabilitation Programs for each client.

The Education of the Handicapped Act Amendments (P.L. 99-457) mandates services for preschoolers. The Part H program is created to assist states in developing a statewide system for early intervention programs for children from birth to three years of age.

Further amendments to the Rehabilitation Act (P.L. 99-506) include consideration for rehabilitative technology services for people with disabilities along with a definition of rehabilitative technology. The legislation also establishes the National Institute of Disability and Rehabilitation Research (NIDRR) from the former National Institute of Handicapped Research (HIHR). Within its mission, the NIDRR supports major research activities, including Rehabilitation Research Engineering Centers (RERCs). RERCs conduct research and development to advance technology and science to solve rehabilitation problems and remove environmental barriers. Each center is affiliated with one or more institutions of higher education or nonprofit organizations.

1987

Speech recognition on computers reaches more than 20,000 words, and Dragon Systems unveils its JAWS screen reader and Naturally Speaking software, which recognizes normal human speech. The possibility for people to activate a computer through speech reaches new heights, making it a realistic tool for oral and written communication.

The U.S. Department of Education establishes the Technology, Educational Media, and Materials Program, with a strategic agenda to drive future planning and priorities in the area of technology.

1988

Flipper, a DOS-based screen reader, is developed by Omnichron of Berkeley, California. Originally designed by John Stephen Smith and Cynthia Lowe for Smith's wife, who was blind, Flipper allows for efficient navigation through documents and books on the computer.

The Technology-Related Assistance for Individuals with Disabilities Act (P.L. 100-407), also known as the Tech Act, recognizes that individuals of all ages with disabilities need special equipment known as assistive technology (AT) to perform better and more independently. The law authorizes funding to states to create statewide systems of technological assistance to meet those needs. It also provides the official federal definitions of AT and AT services.

The first version of ZoomText, a screen magnifier for Microsoft Windows, is released. The software helps individuals with vision loss access the computer. In the future, newer and improved versions are developed.

1989

Matching Person and Technology (MPT) is published by Dr. Marcia Scherer. The model for assessing and matching people to the appropriate technology that is satisfying for the user and caregivers is important. The premise is that MPT makes technology less likely to be abandoned.

1990

P.L. 101-336, the Americans with Disabilities Act (ADA), extends Section 504 of the Rehabilitation Act (P.L. 93-112) requiring equal access and reasonable accommodations in employment to both public and private sectors.

P.L. 101-476, the Education of the Handicapped Act Amendments, renames the law the Individuals with Disabilities Education Act (IDEA). It expands existing programs and services, defines assistive technology devices and services, and adds autism and traumatic brain injury to the list of categories of children and youth eligible for special education services.

The Developmental Disabilities Assistance and Bill of Rights Act (P.L. 101-496), promotes community acceptance and inclusion for all people with developmental disabilities and provides funds to state protection and advocacy agencies for people with disabilities.

The Computer/Electronic Accommodations Program (CAP) is established and provides assistive technology and services to people with disabilities who are employed in federal jobs. CAP increases access and removes barriers to employment opportunities by covering the costs of assistive technology and accommodations.

1991

P.L. 102-119, the Individuals with Disabilities Education Act (IDEA), is signed into law. It extends assistive technology (AT) devices and service definitions to education and mandates that educational programs are responsible for providing AT devices and services if they are needed for the child's education.

1992

P.L. 102-119, the Individuals with Disabilities Education Act Amendments, addresses the Part H (Infants and Toddlers with Disabilities) Program.

P.L. 102-569, the Rehabilitation Act Amendments, are signed into law. The legislation defines rehabilitation technology as "rehabilitation engineering, assistive technology devices and services" and mandates rehabilitation technology as a primary benefit to be included in the clients' individual plans.

Assistive Technology and the IEP is published by RESNA and is a first resource for AT in the schools. The authors define assistive technology devices and services and provide information on how to incorporate assistive technology into an Individualized Education Plan (IEP). In addition, some information on funding sources for assistive technology is included.

1993

The National Institutes of Health (NIH) establish a research plan for the National Center for Medical Rehabilitation Research (NCMRR). A philosophy and framework for research direction related to AT devices and interventions is included. Assistive technology is now a nationally recognized research area.

1994

Myna, a talking handheld computing device for the blind, is introduced.

The introduction of OT FACT (Occupational Therapy Functional Assessment Compilation Tool) software creates a means to standardize the collection of assistive technology assessment data and outcomes data. It isolates assistive technology data within the data elements, furthering the importance of considering AT needs in assessing people with disabilities.

The American Medical Association publishes *Guidelines for the Use of AT*, including evaluation, referral, and prescription. The guidelines are intended to help primary-care physicians efficiently and effectively serve their patients with disabilities.

1995

The U.S. Department of Education creates Regional Education Technology Centers (RETC) to assist in the implementation of technology in public schools.

1996

RESNA publishes a journal dedicated to AT outcomes. Lawrence Trachtman's editorial states that a methodology for measuring and reporting outcomes on AT is needed, bringing national attention to a focus on AT outcomes research and development.

RESNA offers the Assistive Technology Practitioner (ATP) credential examination for the first time.

The Telecommunications Act (P.L. 104-104) requires that telecommunication systems/devices be accessible for people with disabilities and mandates that funding for telecommunication be available to schools and libraries.

1997

P.L. 105-17, the Individuals with Disabilities Education Act Amendments (IDEA), is enacted. The language strengthens the existing law and emphasizes the need to better educate students with disabilities so that they can achieve at the level of peers who do not have disabilities. Included among the law's requirements is one ensuring access to the general curriculum.

National Cash Register Corporation (NCR) develops the first Audio ATM for people who are blind and partially sighted to have access to automated banking. This new development provides accessibility to those who cannot read or write as well.

RESNA publishes *Guidelines for Knowledge and Skills for Provision of the Specialty Technology,* a resource for practitioners. The areas of focus include computer access and control; augmentative and alternative communication; job accommodations; and seating and mobility.

The Association of Assistive Technology Act Programs (ATAP) is established as a member organization. Its mission is to improve the effectiveness of statewide AT programs and promote and facilitate a national network of AT programs.

1998

On August 7 President Bill Clinton signs the Rehabilitation Act Amendments of 1998 into law. The legislation strengthens Section 508 of the Rehabilitation Act, requiring access to electronic and information technology in all federal agencies.

P.L. 105-394, the Assistive Technology Act, is signed into law, extending funding of the 1988 Tech Act to assist states in promoting awareness of AT, as well as in providing technical assistance, outreach, and interagency coordination. The grants now go to all 50 states and all U.S. territories.

The National Assistive Technology Technical Assistance Partnership (NATTAP) is formed to support and provide technical assistance and training to the statewide AT programs, the Alternative Finance programs, and the Protection and Advocacy programs. It is funded under the AT Act of 1998 and its 2004 amendments.

P.L. 98-199, the Education of the Handicapped Act Amendments, is reauthorized. The legislation emphasizes services to facilitate school-to-work transition, establishes regional parent training and information centers, and provides funding for early intervention and early childhood special education projects.

The Assistive Technology Industry Association (ATIA), a not-for-profit membership organization of manufacturers, sellers, and providers of technology-based assistive devices and/or services, is founded. Its mission is to represent its members and ensure that the best possible products and services are made available to people with disabilities.

Nokia releases the LPS-1 Loopset, which allows people who have a hearing loss and use hearing aids to use a mobile phone. This is the first technology of its type and opens communication options for those with hearing impairments.

Quality Indicators for AT (QIAT) is a grassroots effort that begins in 1998 with a purpose to develop indicators of effective practices, evaluation tools for continuous improvement, and resources for collaborators. This evolves into a nationwide effort with over a thousand members.

WYNN, a new literacy software tool, comes on the market. By simultaneously highlighting text as it is spoken, making printed text more understandable, this technology helps those with limited English proficiency, reading difficulties, and attention disorders.

Blazie Engineering announces the Type Lite, a portable note taker with a QWERTY keyboard, speech output, and a 40-cell Braille display.

1999

The World Wide Web Consortium (W3C), an international community, begins working to develop Web standards for rich and accessible communication and interaction for all. W3C's mission is "to lead the Web to its full potential," which involves participation, sharing knowledge, and thereby building trust on a global scale.

The National Institute on Disability and Rehabilitation Research (NIDRR) issues a new long-range plan that emphasizes research and development in the area of assistive technology. This opens the door for more grant opportunities to conduct research projects on all aspects of AT.

The first ATIA conference occurs in Orlando. In the years to come, conferences are held annually and then biannually, with one in Florida and one in Chicago.

2000

The U.S Department of Education gives the National Assistive Technology Research Institute (NATRI) funds to conduct research on outcomes in assistive technology.

2001

President George W. Bush signs major education-reform legislation known as the No Child Left Behind Act. An updated version of the 1965 Elementary and Secondary Education Act (ESEA), it now addresses services and expectations for the disability community and holds schools accountable for the achievement of students with disabilities.

The Commission on Accreditation of Rehabilitation Facilities (CARF International) issues the *Employment and Community Services Standards Manual*. New in this set of standards is a section titled assistive technology services.

The ATOMS project (Assistive Technology Outcomes Measurement Study) is funded for five years by the National Institute on Disability and Rehabilitation Research (NIDRR). The purpose is to determine how to objectively assess the use of assistive technology.

With the unanimous endorsement of the 54th World Health Assembly, the International Classification of Functioning, Disability, and Health (ICF) is adopted as the framework for describing and measuring health and disability. In the World Health Organization (WHO), the ICF framework is used in the Multi-Country Survey Study in 2000/2001 and the World Health Survey Program in 2002/2003 to measure health status of the general population in 71 countries. Disability attributes are considered universally as something that anyone can experience and not a separate population group.

On February 1 President Bush announces the New Freedom Initiative (NFI). As a nationwide effort to remove barriers to community living for people of all ages with disabilities and long-term illnesses, it includes consideration for technology to improve access to independence.

On December 21 the Access Board, an independent federal agency devoted to accessibility for people with disabilities, issues accessibility standards for information technology as required in Section 508 of the Rehabilitation Act.

2002

The Professional Standards Board in Assistive and Rehabilitation Technology establishes the Rehabilitation Engineering Technologist (RET) certificate examination process. RESNA oversees this program.

2004

P.L. 108-364, the Assistive Technology Act Amendments, implements reporting requirements that increase accountability of the statewide AT programs. The focus is on how people with disabilities are benefiting from increased awareness, training, and acquisition of assistive technology.

2008

The Defense Department includes assistive technology in the assessment and recovery process for Wounded Warriors. The Computer/Electronic Accommodations Program (CAPTEC) offers Wounded Warriors assistive technologies and training to help them cope with life's daily tasks throughout all phases of their personal recovery.

2010

The U.S. Department of Education funds RESNA to implement a new national technical assistance program for the statewide assistive technology programs. The CATALYST Project, a collaboration between RESNA and the Neighborhood Legal Association, has a mission to provide technical assistance and training to support the implementation of the Assistive Technology Act of 2004, as amended.

The Twenty-First Century Communications and Video Accessibility Act (CVAA) is signed into law by President Barack Obama. The CVAA is considered the most significant piece of accessibility legislation since the passage of the Americans with Disabilities Act in 1990. The CVAA modernizes existing communications laws to ensure that people with disabilities are able to share fully in the economic, social, and civic benefits of broadband and other 21st-century communication technologies.

On December 7, Chairman Julius Genachowski announces the establishment of the Emergency Access Advisory Committee (EAAC), which is required by CVAA. The purpose of the EAAC is to determine the most effective and efficient technologies and methods by which to enable access to Next Generation 911 emergency services by individuals with disabilities.

Section 255 of the Communications Act requires telecommunications and interconnected Voice over Internet Protocol (VoIP) manufacturers to provide access. Before its passage, people with disabilities often did not have full access to the benefits of rapid technological changes in advanced communications, including wireless capable of accessing the Internet, sending e-mails or text messages, and enabling video conversations.

Four

Biographies of Key Contributors in the Field

Cathy Bodine, Lorrie Harkness, and Maureen Melonis

Many individuals have made significant contributions to the invention, development, and promotion of assistive technology for persons with disabilities. The biographical sketches in this chapter, presented in alphabetical order, profile some of those individuals and their contributions.

David Abraham (1896–1978)

Inventor of the Perkins Brailler

David Abraham was born in Liverpool, England, in 1896. He served in the Royal Flying Corps during World War I, and then joined his family's stair rail manufacturing business, where he displayed an affinity for machinery design. He immigrated to the United States in the late 1920s, shortly before the onset of the Great Depression. The dire economic conditions forced Abraham to take work as a manual laborer despite his skills as a craftsman and mechanic.

In the early 1930s, Abraham was assigned to a road repair crew in Watertown, Massachusetts, that was carrying out work near the Perkins School for the Blind, the first school of its kind in the United States. Founded in 1832, the school's past students had included Helen Keller. On impulse Abraham approached the campus and asked for work. He was rewarded with a position as an instructor in the school's manual training department (he also worked in the maintenance department during the summer).

In the mid-1930s, the director of the school, Dr. Gabriel Farrell, approached Abraham with a request to try his hand at designing a new braillewriter—a device similar to a typewriter for writing in Braille. Vexed by the limitations of the Braille writing machines being produced at that time by Perkins and other manufacturers, Farrell felt that research into new design possibilities was overdue. Abraham promptly accepted the challenge, which rekindled his dormant mechanical design talents. Over the next several years Farrell worked closely with Dr. Edward J. Waterhouse, the assistant manager of the school's publishing arm, to make sure that his design would meet the needs of Braille users. In addition, Abraham devoted countless hours to working on the project in his home workshop in nearby Waltham.

In November 1939, Abraham unveiled his first prototype to Waterhouse, who responded positively. Abraham returned to his workshop to further hone his invention, and in 1941 he presented his device to the school's trustees. They were dazzled by Abraham's complex and durable but easy-to-use design, which featured a key corresponding to each of the six dots of the Braille code, as well as individual keys for spaces, backspaces, and line spaces. After wartime manufacturing restrictions were lifted in 1945, the school invested heavily in the new-generation "Perkins Brailler." The first of Abraham's machines became commercially available in 1951, and the device quickly became known among people with blindness as the finest braillewriter on the market. It retained its popularity for the next half-century, even after the development of various electronic Braille devices and translation software. Often cited as the Braille equivalent of a pen and paper, it is also heavily utilized in developing nations. Abraham's design remained intact until 2008, when the Perkins School released a new version, dubbed the Next Generation Perkins Brailler.

Abraham remained with the Perkins School until 1961, when he retired as head of the school's industrial arts department. He spent his retirement years in Florida, where he devoted much of his free time to sailing. He died in 1978 at the age of eighty-two.

Further Reading

French, K. (2004). *Perkins School for the Blind.* Charleston, SC: Arcadia Publishing.
Seymour-Ford, J. (2002). History of the Perkins Brailler. Retrieved from http://
    www.perkins.org/resources/curricular/literacy/brailler-history.html
Waterhouse, E. J. (1975). *History of the Howe Press of Perkins School for the Blind*
    Watertown, MA: Howe Press of Perkins School for the Blind.

Bruce Baker

Inventor of the Minspeak augmentative communication system

Bruce Roland Baker developed a passion for language at an early age. He recalled picking up a Latin textbook at age six and being enthralled by the idea of learning a language that had once been the dominant language of the Roman Empire. A top student, Baker earned a bachelor's degree in Latin with a minor in Greek in 1967 from Wabash College in Crawfordsville, Indiana. He then continued his education at Middlebury College in Vermont, where he received a master's degree in French language and literature in 1976.

Baker's pioneering work in symbol systems and language representation in augmentative communication/assistive technology began in the late 1970s, when he began work on a doctoral program in modern linguistics and language teaching at Middlebury. His research brought him into contact with people who had a variety of communication disabilities. These encounters inspired Baker to develop an augmentative communication system that would be more effective than the primitive ones currently available to people with severe communication disabilities. In 1980 he unveiled the Minspeak system for people with physical obstacles to writing, talking, and hand signing modes of communication. This patented visual language system, based on the use of commonly recognized picture icons in various combinations, was devised by Baker so that it could be used by a person to communicate a wide range of ideas and information, from the simple to the complex.

In 1982 Baker founded Semantic Compaction Systems, which owns the copyright to the Minspeak system and many other forms of intellectual property developed by Baker in the assistive technology field over the years. In 1983, a commercially available Minspeak computer program was unveiled at the American Speech-Language-Hearing Association

(ASHA) convention in Cincinnati, Ohio. Since that time the Minspeak approach has evolved to address the needs of adults and children with a wide range of communication impairments. Minspeak computer interface programs are available today in English, Spanish, French, Italian, German, Japanese, and Swedish.

In addition to his Minspeak work, Baker has been recognized for his contributions to United Cerebral Palsy, the International Society for Augmentative and Alternative Communication, and other humanitarian organizations. In 1993, he founded the nonprofit organization Support Helps Others Use Technology (SHOUT), which studies employment issues for people with significant communication impairments. He also serves as an adjunct associate professor at the University of Pittsburgh's School of Health and Rehabilitation Sciences.

Further Reading

About Bruce Baker (n.d.). Retrieved from http://www.minspeak.com/students/AboutBruceBaker.php

Baker, B. R. (2009). Minspeak history. Retrieved from http://www.minspeak.com/HistoryofMinspeak.php

Baker, B. R., Hill, K., & Devylder, R. (2000). Core vocabulary is the same across environments. Center on Disabilities Technology and Persons with Disabilities Conference 2000. Retrieved from http://www.csun.edu/cod/conf/2000/proceedings/0259Baker.htm

Graham A. Barden (1896–1967)

Congressman who co-authored the Barden-LaFollette Rehabilitation Act

Graham Arthur Barden was born in Turkey Township, Sampson County, North Carolina, on September 25, 1896. He served in the U.S. Navy during World War I, and in 1920 he earned a law degree from the University of North Carolina at Chapel Hill. Admitted to the bar that same year, he promptly opened a law practice in New Bern, North Carolina.

In 1932 Barden was elected to the state House of Representatives as a Democrat. Two years later, he ran for a seat in the U.S. Congress. He narrowly defeated his district's incumbent Democrat in the primary, then cruised to victory in the general election. This triumph paved the way for the first of thirteen consecutive terms that Barden would serve in Washington, D.C., as the representative of North Carolina's Third Congressional District.

Barden became a powerful and influential congressman during his long tenure in Washington. He served as chairman of committees on education and labor issues at various points in his career, and he was a high-profile supporter of Franklin D. Roosevelt's early New Deal policies. During World War II, Barden was able to use his influence to bring Camp Davis, Camp Lejeune, and Cherry Point Air Station to his home district.

Barden also helped revolutionize government policies regarding the rehabilitation and assistance to individuals with disabilities when he teamed with Senator Robert M. LaFollette Jr. (R-WI) to craft the Barden-LaFollette Rehabilitation Act. This legislation, which passed Congress in June 1943, greatly strengthened the 1920 Vocational Rehabilitation Act. It established the federal government as a full administrative and financial partner with individual states in efforts to rehabilitate and provide vocational training to employable adults with disabilities, including individuals with blindness, amputations, and mental illness. The act gave state rehabilitation agencies the financial certainty and administrative support they needed to plan and organize their work on a systematic basis.

Passage of the 1943 act was such a transformative event that it became known as the Magna Carta of the blind, according to scholar Frances Koestler. "Before 1943, if a man lost a leg, a rehabilitation agency had to train him for a job that could be done by a one-legged man," she explained. "After 1943, the agency had the funds to buy an artificial limb and turn the man into a two-legged worker. The same analogy applied to clients blinded by cataracts or other medically correctable eye defects."

By the time World War II ended in 1945, Barden's political views were growing more conservative. He played a significant role in the creation and passage of the 1947 Taft-Hartley Act, which placed heavy restrictions on union organizing. He also became a vocal opponent of federal "interference" in state public education, and he was a signatory to the so-called Southern Manifesto, which condemned the Supreme Court's landmark 1954 *Brown v. Board of Education* anti-segregation ruling as unconstitutional. Barden retired in 1960, and he died in New Bern on January 29, 1967.

Further Reading

Koestler, F. A. (1976). *The unseen minority: A social history of blindness in the United States.* New York, NY: American Foundation for the Blind.

Puryear, E. (1979). *Graham A. Barden, conservative Carolina congressman.* Buie's Creek, NC: Campbell University Press.

Schultz, W. (n.d.). Graham A. Barden (1896–1967). Retrieved from http://www .northcarolinahistory.org/encyclopedia/416/entry

Alexander Graham Bell (1847–1922)

American inventor of the telephone and teacher for deaf people

Alexander Graham Bell was born on March 3, 1847 in Edinburgh, Scotland. He is universally known as the inventor of the telephone, but it was his research and passion for helping deaf people communicate that made the invention possible. That passion developed very early in his life. It was inspired by his father, Alexander Melville Bell, an internationally known expert in vocal physiology who developed the Visible Speech system to help deaf people learn to speak, and his mother, Eliza Grace Symonds Bell, a painter and musician who was deaf.

By age 16 Bell was already attending Edinburgh University. He also spent time at University College in London helping his father teach deaf students. While there, Bell met Charles Wheatstone, who had patented England's first electronic telegraph, and became fascinated with the developing technology of sound transmission. He went on to study phonetics and physiology and spent some time teaching at a school for the deaf in South Kensington. Soon after, however, tragedy struck the Bell family when both of Alexander's brothers died from tuberculosis. With Alexander battling the disease as well, in 1870 his parents decided to move to what they hoped would be a better climate in Canada. Alexander continued on to Boston to teach at the Sarah Fuller School for the Deaf, and in 1873 he took a position as professor of vocal physiology at Boston University's School of Oratory.

By 1874 Bell had developed his basic concept for a telephone, but he needed someone to help him build it. That year he met Thomas Watson, a Boston machinist, and they partnered to work on Bell's design. After a series of failed experiments, Bell was finally able to successfully transmit the first telephone message. He received a U.S. patent for his invention on March 7, 1876, and the following year he formed the Bell Telephone Company.

Soon after, Bell married one of his former students, Mabel Hubbard, and they had two children. They traveled to Europe to promote the telephone, and in 1880 he won the Volta Prize from the French government in recognition of his invention. With the money earned from that prize, he returned to the United States and built the Volta Laboratory in Washington, D.C., where he continued his research and inventing. He also returned to his studies of hearing impairment, and in 1887 he founded the Volta Bureau, which was dedicated to increasing knowledge of deafness. In 1890 Bell was elected president of the American Association for the Promotion and Teaching of Speech to the Deaf (AAPTSD), and in 1908 the AAPTSD merged with the Volta Bureau.

Bell died on August 2, 1922, at his summer home in Baddeck, Nova Scotia. While he is remembered primarily for his invention of the telephone, his legacy as a lifelong advocate for people who are deaf or hard of hearing was confirmed in 1956 when the AAPTSD was renamed the Alexander Graham Bell Association for the Deaf.

Further Reading

Gray, C. (2006). *Reluctant genius: Alexander Graham Bell and the passion for invention.* New York, NY: Arcade Publishing.

Bruce, R. V. (1973). *Bell: Alexander Graham Bell and the conquest of solitude.* Boston, MA: Little, Brown.

David R. Beukelman

Leading researcher in the field of augmentative and alternative communication

David R. Beukelman is a speech-language pathologist who specializes in augmentative and alternative communication (AAC) and communication disorders associated with physical and neurological conditions. His professional affiliations include the Rehabilitation Engineering and Research Center for Communication Enhancement, where he is a partner, and the Institute for Rehabilitation Science and Engineering at Madonna Rehabilitation Hospital in Lincoln, Nebraska, where he is a senior researcher. He is also director of research and education of the Communication Disorders Division of the Munroe/Meyer Institute of Genetics and Rehabilitation in Omaha, Nebraska. In addition, Beukelman is the Barkley Professor of Communication Disorders at the University of Nebraska-Lincoln. His courses of instruction in Lincoln include augmentative and alternative communication, motor speech disorders, and cleft palate.

Beukelman has written widely on augmentative and alternative communication issues over the years. In addition to numerous scholarly articles, his credits as author include *Augmentative and Alternative Communication: Management of Severe Communication Disorders in Children and Adults* (1998) and *Augmentative and Alternative Communication: Supporting Children and Adults with Complex Communication Needs* (2006). He has also served as editor of *Augmentative and Alternative Communication Journal* and has published numerous articles and co-authored several books relating to AAC. Beukelman is a past recipient of the President's Award from the International Society for Augmentative and Alternative Communication.

Further Reading

Beukelman, D. R., & Mirenda, P. (2006). *Augmentative and alternative communication: Supporting children and adults with complex communication needs.* Baltimore, MD: Paul H. Brookes, 2006.

Deane Blazie (1946–)

Entrepreneur and engineer who developed computer devices for people who are blind

Deane Blazie was born in 1946 in Detroit, but he grew up in Kentucky. As a youth he became acquainted with Tim Cranmer, a famous engineer in the assistive technology industry. Cranmer became a mentor to Blazie, who assisted on many of Cranmer's projects in the 1960s.

Blazie graduated from the University of Kentucky with an engineering degree in 1968. He spent the next year and a half working for Western Electric in New Mexico before being drafted into the U.S. Army in 1970. He spent most of his 18 months of military service working for the army's Human Engineering Laboratory, which was devoted to designing military materials in ways that maximize their comfort and utility for soldiers. Blazie later described this experience as a valuable one for designing products "because every time I think about a product feature I would think of my human factors stuff and I would be very conscious of how important that was."

In 1976 Blazie joined with Richard Kramer (a fellow alumnus of the Human Engineering Laboratory) to establish Maryland Computer Services, which specialized in developing products for the blind. In 1986 Blazie formed a new company, Blazie Engineering, where he developed the Braille 'n' Speak, the world's first notetaker with Braille key input and speech or data output. This pocket-sized data organizing and management device, which included note taking, calendar, calculator, and address/contact functions, became very popular among students and professionals with sight impairments after its introduction in 1988. Blazie also helped develop a number of other hardware products for the blind over the next several years, including Braille embossers and refreshable Braille displays.

In 2000 Blazie Engineering merged with Henter/Joyce and Arkenstone, two other companies heavily involved in making products for people with visual impairments. The new company, Freedom Scientific, continues to offer a broad line of assistive technology products for people with learning disabilities and sensory impairments. In 2001 Blazie left Freedom Scientific and retired to Hobe Sound, Florida.

Further Reading

Candela, T. (2004). An oral history interview with Deane Blazie, parts 1–5. Retrieved from http://www.afb.org/Section.asp?SectionID=4&TopicID=456& SubTopicID=232&DocumentID=5452

George W. Bush (1946–)

Forty-third president of the United States, signer of the 2001 Freedom Initiative on Disability

George Walker Bush was born July 6, 1946, in New Haven, Connecticut. He was the oldest son of Barbara and George H.W. Bush, a government official and diplomat who later became the forty-first president of the United States (1989–1993). In 1948 the family moved to Texas, where Bush spent most of his childhood. He received a bachelor's degree in history from Yale University in 1968 and then served as a pilot in the Texas Air National Guard. In 1975 he earned a master's degree in business administration from Harvard Business School.

After graduating from Harvard, Bush settled in Texas where he pursued a variety of ventures in the oil business. In 1989 he assembled a group of investors that purchased the Texas Rangers baseball franchise. He became increasingly involved in state and national politics around this time, and on November 8, 1994, Bush was elected the forty-sixth governor of Texas as a Republican. He won a second four-year term as governor in November 1998. Midway through his second term, Bush decided to run for president of the United States. He won the Republican nomination and faced off against the Democratic nominee, Vice President Al Gore, in the general election in November 2000. Bush narrowly won the election—despite losing the popular vote—after a controversial U.S. Supreme Court decision preserved the Republican's narrow edge in the Electoral College, and he was sworn into office on January 20, 2001. Bush was re-elected over Democratic nominee John Kerry on November 2, 2004, and sworn in for a second term on January 20, 2005.

During his eight-year presidency, Bush's most ambitious program on disability issues was his 2001 Freedom Initiative on Disability, which (1) acknowledged widespread discrimination against persons with disabilities in the United States, and (2) provided for an assortment of policies and programs to address this discrimination and promote the full participation of people with disabilities in American society. Specifically, the initiative included proposals to increase access to assistive and universally designed technology, to expand education opportunities, to ensure full integration into the work force, and to promote increased participation in the daily life of the wider community. The initiative included specific requests for funding—including $1 billion to give people with disabilities greater access to new assistive technologies—and called for full implementation of existing statutes, such as the Ticket to Work and Work Incentives Improvement Act of 1999 and the Individuals with Disabilities Education Act.

The most notable other advance in disability policy during the Bush years came in 2008, when the Americans with Disabilities Act Amendments Act (ADAAA) was passed by both houses of Congress and signed into law by Bush. This legislation significantly broadened the scope of protection intended by Congress to be available under the 1990 Americans with Disabilities Act. A direct response to Supreme Court decisions that had limited the scope of the ADA, the ADAAA expanded the protections of the original ADA to include more individuals with less severe impairments and emphasized the obligations of employers to provide "reasonable" workplace accommodations for workers with disabilities.

Further Reading

Bush, G. W. (2010). *Decision points*. New York, NY: Crown.

The President's New Freedom Initiative: The 2007 progress report (2007). Retrieved from http://georgewbush-whitehouse.archives.gov/infocus/newfreedom/newfreedom-report-2007.html

Zelizer, J. E. (Ed.). (2010). *The presidency of George W. Bush: A first historical assessment*. Princeton, NJ: Princeton University Press.

Dinah Cohen (1953–)

Director of the Department of Defense's
Computer/Electronic Accommodations Program (CAP)

The daughter of Holocaust survivors, Dinah Cohen struggled with a congenital heart disease at a young age. This experience helped set her on a career path of rehabilitation and advocacy work for people with disabilities. "Growing up with my own disabilities, I am inspired to make sure others can succeed in their chosen careers as I have," she explained. Cohen received a bachelor's degree in social science/elementary education from Russell Sage College in Troy, New York, in the early 1970s. She then went on to earn a master's degree in counseling psychology (with a concentration in rehabilitation counseling) from the State University of New York.

Cohen began her career as a rehabilitation counselor by visiting injured soldiers at Veterans Administration and military hospitals. In 1990 she was hired as the first director of the U.S. Department of Defense's Computer/Electronic Accommodations Program (CAP). The CAP program was designed initially to provide training and assistive technology to wounded veterans to increase their opportunities for employment. Under the CAP process, medical centers identify the assistive technology needs of veterans with disabilities, then train them in the use of this equipment as the veterans undergo rehabilitation. Examples of assistive technology provided through CAP include specialized voice recognition and screen magnification software, assistive listening devices, computer-based applications to help with memory loss, Braille terminals, and specialized keyboards for people who have lost the use of their hands. Another important resource developed by Cohen is the CAP Technology Evaluation Center, an assessment and demonstration facility which serves as a resource for senior federal government workers interested in learning more about assistive technology options.

CAP was initially crafted solely for Pentagon employees, but under Cohen's dynamic leadership CAP expanded its mission in 2000 to provide assistive technology services to employees with disabilities in more than 65 federal government agencies. It also has become an important resource for military service personnel returning from Iraq and Afghanistan with debilitating injuries. By the close of 2009 the program—the largest assistive technology program in the world—had provided assistance to an estimated 90,000 individuals.

Cohen frequently speaks around the world on disability policy, assistive technology, and accessibility issues. In 2007 she received the Service to America Medal for Citizen Service. One year later, CAP was honored with the 2008 President's Quality Award for Management Excellence, which is the highest award given to executive branch agencies.

Further Reading

Partnership for Public Service (2007). 2007 Citizen Services Medal recipient: Dinah F. B. Cohen. Retrieved from http://servicetoamericamedals.org/SAM/recipients/profiles/csm07_cohen.shtml

Partnership for Public Service (2009, October 26). Dinah Cohen: Helping wounded veterans re-enter the workforce. *Washington Post*. Retrieved from http://www.washingtonpost.com/wp-dyn/content/article/2009/10/26/AR2009102600529.html

Albert Cook

Researcher in augmentative technology and communication

Albert Cook attributes his pioneering work in assistive technology and rehabilitation to his own family's experiences. When his son Brian was born with a severe intellectual disability in the late 1970s, Cook left a promising career in electrical engineering—a career grounded in academic training at the University of Colorado (where he received a bachelor's degree in electrical engineering)—to pursue work in the assistive technology field. He subsequently earned a master's degree in bioengineering and a doctorate from the University of Wyoming.

Cook began his academic career at California State University, Sacramento, where he founded the Biomedical Engineering Graduate Program and co-directed the Assistive Device Center. He moved to Canada in 1994 to take the position of dean of the faculty of rehabilitation medicine at the University of Alberta. He served in that capacity for the next 14 years, helping to establish the faculty as a world reference in research, development, and service provision in rehabilitation medicine and assistive technology. From 2000 to 2007 he also served as chair of the Health Sciences Council.

Since 2007 Cook has been a professor in the Department of Speech Pathology and Audiology and special advisor to the provost at the University of Alberta. He has also served in various positions with the Institute of Electrical and Electronic Engineers, the Engineering in

Medicine and Biology Society, the American Society for Engineering Education, the Biomedical Engineering Society, the International Society for Augmentative and Alternative Communication, and the Association for the Advancement of Medical Instrumentation. In 1997–1998 he served as president of the Rehabilitation Engineering and Assistive Technology Society of North America (RESNA), a leading professional society for assistive technology practitioners in North America.

Cook's research interests have included augmentative and alternative communication, biomedical instrumentation, and assistive technology design, development, and evaluation. In recent years he has focused much of his research on robotics that provide for the assessment and development of cognitive and linguistic skills in young children who have severe disabilities. He has been invited as a keynote speaker to many international conferences on assistive technology. Cook is also the co-author (with Janice Polgar) of the popular textbook *Cook and Hussey's Assistive Technologies: Principles and Practice,* as well as the author of numerous chapters in rehabilitation and biomedical engineering texts, monographs, peer reviewed papers, and conference proceedings. In 2010 Cook received the SIGACCESS Award for Outstanding Contribution to Computing and Accessibility, an international award in recognition of his lifelong dedication to the research and development of assistive devices and computing technology for persons with disabilities.

Further Reading

Cook, A. (2010). The future of assistive technologies: A time of promise and apprehension. Proceedings of the 12th International ACM SIGACCESS Conference on Computers and Accessibility, New York.

Cook, A., & Polgar, J. (2007). *Cook and Hussey's assistive technologies: Principles and practice.* St. Louis, MO: Mosby Elsevier.

Gray, H. (2010, June 29). Speech professor Al Cook receives international computing award. Retrieved from http://www.uofaweb.ualberta.ca/spa/news.cfm?story=99501

Tim Cranmer (1925–2001)

*Activist and inventor of assistive devices
for people with visual impairments*

Terence V. "Tim" Cranmer was born on February 3, 1925, in Louisville, Kentucky. He was blind from childhood and had only limited schooling, completing the sixth grade at the Kentucky School for the Blind. As a young adult he sold plastic jewelry, worked at Kentucky Industries for the Blind, and supported himself as a piano technician. In 1952 he began working for the Kentucky Division of Rehabilitation Services for the Blind (later known as the Kentucky Department for the Blind). He rose through the ranks of this state agency and played a pivotal role in establishing and supervising a technology division within the department. Cranmer also became known from the 1960s forward for his strong activism as a member of the National Federation of the Blind. He served as the first vice president of the NFB's Kentucky affiliate and established the federation's first state-level department devoted to computer issues for members.

Cranmer also developed a number of important inventions for people with visual impairments during these decades. His inventions ranged from early electronic Braille printers and computer screen readers to the so-called "Cranmer Abacus." This device, which Cranmer unveiled in 1962, modified the traditional Chinese abacus so that people who were blind could use it for arithmetic problems. He also developed audio/ tactile Braille displays for use with clocks, stopwatches, and clinical system monitors, and he created a Braille font with tactile graphics for use with the Pixelmaster.

In 1982 Cranmer retired from the Kentucky Department for the Blind and embarked on two ambitious new projects. The first was to establish a research and development arm of the National Federation of the Blind. He also founded the International Braille Research Center in Kentucky in 1994. Even while engaged in these time-consuming projects, however, Cranmer continued to pursue his love of invention and his interest in assistive technology. He contributed, for example, to the electronic circuitry and design of both the Braille 'n' Speak and Braille Lite data organizers for people with visual impairments. Cranmer died on November 15, 2001.

Further Reading

Hanse, B. (2002). Louisville loses blind inventor and advocate: Tim Cranmer made the unseen visible. Retrieved from http://www.nfbky.org/cranmer.php

Kenrick, D. (2002, January). Tim Cranmer: One of our great pioneers. *Access News*, 3(1), Retrieved from http://www.afb.org/afbpress/pub.asp?Doc ID=aw0301news

Harvey Fletcher (1884–1981)

American researcher in communication acoustics

Harvey Fletcher was born on September 11, 1884, in Provo, Utah, to Charles and Elizabeth Fletcher. In 1908 he married Lorena Chipman, with whom he eventually had seven children. Two years after Lorena's death in 1967, he married her sister, Fern Eyring.

Fletcher earned a Bachelor of Science degree from Brigham Young University in 1907 and a Ph.D. in physics from the University of Chicago in 1911, graduating summa cum laude. While at the University of Chicago he helped Robert A. Millikan discover a method for measuring the charge of an electron. This scientific breakthrough earned Millikan a Nobel Prize in 1923 and became the foundation for Fletcher's brilliant career as a researcher and inventor.

After completing his Ph.D., Fletcher went back to Brigham Young University as chair of the school's physics department. He remained there until 1916, when he took a position at the Western Electric Company of New York, working in sound research. He later moved on to Bell Laboratories, where he worked as the company's director of physical research until 1949. During his time at Bell Labs, Fletcher developed a passion for finding a way to accurately produce, transmit, and record sound. He played a major role in a number of important auditory discoveries and inventions in such realms as sound motion pictures, high-fidelity recording, improved telephone transmission, sonar, the artificial larynx, and the first electronic hearing aid. Some scholars have even described him as the single greatest intellectual force in the development of present-day communication acoustics and telephony.

Fletcher was one of the founders (and the first president) of the Acoustical Society of America. He also served as president of the American Society for the Hard of Hearing, and he was a member of the National Hearing Division Committee of Medical Sciences and an honorary member of the American Speech and Hearing Society.

In 1949 Fletcher left Bell Labs for a teaching position at Columbia University. In 1952 he returned to his beloved alma mater, Brigham Young University, where he oversaw research and helped to set up the Department of Engineering and the College of Physical and Engineering Sciences. In 1960 Fletcher returned to studying acoustics, researching musical tones and their expression through instrumentation. By the time of his death in 1981, he had acquired over 40 patents for acoustical devices, published more than 60 scientific papers, and received numerous honors and awards, including membership in the National Academy of Sciences and a Presidential Citation from Harry S. Truman.

Further Reading

Allen, J. B. (1996, April). Harvey Fletcher's role in the creation of communication acoustics. *Journal of the Acoustical Society of America, 99*(4), 1825–1839.
Fletcher, S. H. (1992). *Harvey Fletcher, 1884–1981: A biographical memoir.* Washington, DC: National Academy of Sciences. Retrieved from http://books.nap.edu/html/biomems/hfletcher.pdf

Frank Hall (1841–1911)

Educator of blind students and inventor of the Hall Braillewriter

Frank Haven Hall was born on February 9, 1841, in Mechanic Falls, Maine. When the Civil War came he served as a member of the Twenty-Third Regiment, Maine Volunteer Infantry. Following the war he taught at Towle Academy in Maine. In 1866 he moved west and landed in Illinois, where he became a public school principal in several towns and villages, including Earlville, West Aurora, Sugar Grove, Petersburgh, and Waukegan. At various periods he also supplemented his administrator's salary by working as a postmaster and a township treasurer and clerk, and for a time he owned a creamery and a lumber yard.

In 1890 Hall was named superintendent of the Illinois School for the Blind in Jacksonville, Illinois. A discerning and empathetic administrator, Hall expressed great dissatisfaction with the slow and cumbersome writing resources—a slate and hand-held stylus—available to his blind students. He promptly decided to invent a typewriter for people who were blind—a Braillewriter—that would make it easier for them to correspond and publish Braille materials in mass quantities. With the assistance of local gunsmith Gustav Sieber, within two years Hall developed a working model capable of typing raised Braille dots on standard-sized paper. He introduced his mechanical writing invention on May 27, 1892. Within a matter of weeks, his invention—for which he did not seek a patent—was being manufactured by the Harrison & Seifried Company in Chicago. Hall's Braillewriter, which he soon adapted to a form that could print multiple copies (the Braille Stereotyper), had a revolutionary impact on people with blindness. It galvanized the mass production of books and other materials in Braille and gave blind students an important communication tool for their continued education and future professional careers.

Hall also became an effective advocate for the rights of his students during this period. When school authorities in Chicago weighed whether to establish a boarding school for blind students in the late 1890s, Hall criticized the idea as one that reflected ignorance of the true capacities of students with sight impairments. He subsequently convinced the administrators to establish day classes for the students instead. As a result, the first public school day class for blind students was initiated in Chicago in 1900, with one of Hall's teachers as supervisor.

In 1902 Hall concluded his service with the Illinois School for the Blind. He spent the next nine years as superintendent of the Farmers' Institute of Illinois, an organization concerned with agricultural education. He died in 1911 in Aurora, Illinois.

Further Reading

Farrell, G. (1956). *The story of blindness*. Cambridge, MA: Harvard University Press.
Henrickson, W. B. (1956). The three lives of Frank H. Hall. *Journal of the Illinois State Historical Society, 44*, 271–293.

Jim Halliday

Maker of assistive technology products for people with sight impairments and other disabilities

Jim Halliday's long and successful career in the assistive technology (AT) industry began in the early 1970s, when he was employed in media production for a community college in Cupertino, California. One of his projects involved putting together a multimedia presentation to help convince state lawmakers to approve additional funding for services for students with disabilities. The finished product attracted the attention of executives at Telesensory Systems Inc. (TCI), one of the nation's leading producers of high-tech products for people with blindness or other visual impairments. Halliday produced several documentary/sales films for TCI before joining the company. By the time he left TCI in 1987, he was the company's worldwide sales and marketing director.

Halliday's departure from TCI was noted by Russell Smith, a top executive with the New Zealand-based Wormald International Sensory Aids (later Pulse Data International-PDI). Smith and Halliday agreed to co-found a new company, which they called HumanWare. "At the time, every other company in the industry had names like 'systems' or 'engineering' or 'scientific,' but none seemed to focus on people," said Halliday, who served as president and CEO of the new company. "For me, it was all about people. I believed that you could only produce the best technology if you put people first, so we named our new company HumanWare."

Over the next two decades HumanWare became a major player in the AT industry on the strength of an array of products for blind people, including note-taking products, Braille displays, and closed-circuit television (CCTV)-based video magnifiers. In 2000 the company was acquired by Tieman (now Optalec), a major manufacturer of electronic equipment for people with visual impairments. Conflicts over business strategy and priorities with Tieman executives resulted in Halliday's ouster in March 2001, but a few months later Pulse Data bought the company and Halliday was reinstated (along with several HumanWare staff members who had resigned in protest of his dismissal).

Halliday served HumanWare as president and CEO until late 2003. He remained in a leadership position with the company for the next several years, but he also spent this time laying the groundwork for retirement. In 2005, for example, he and his wife, Karen, established a vineyard in Oregon. Halliday finally retired from HumanWare in March 2008, but he continued his affiliation with the company on a consulting basis. He also remained an active presence in the assistive technology industry, both as a speaker at industry gatherings and as an ambassador for people with AT needs.

Further Reading

Kendrick, D. (2001, September). The human touch in HumanWare. *AccessWorld*, 2(5). Retrieved from http://www.afb.org/afbpress/pub.asp?DocID=aw020503

Tom Harkin (1939–)

Politician who played a leading role in developing and passing the Americans with Disabilities Act and other legislation related to disabilities

Tom Harkin was born in Cumming, Iowa, on November 19, 1939. The son of an Iowa coal miner father and a Slovenian immigrant mother, he still lives in the house where he was born. He learned sign language at an early age because his brother, Frank, was deaf. A graduate of Dowling High School in Des Moines, Iowa, Harkin attended Iowa State University on a Navy ROTC scholarship, earning a degree in government and economics in 1962. He then served in the Navy as an active-duty jet pilot from 1962 to 1967, during which time his postings included Japan and Guantanamo Bay, Cuba. In 1968 he married Ruth Raduenz, with whom he had two children.

Harkin's career in politics began in 1969, when he joined the Washington, D.C., staff of Neal Smith, a Democratic congressman from Iowa. He also continued his schooling, and in 1972 he graduated from Catholic University of America Law School in Washington, D.C. Harkin then returned to Iowa, where he waged an unsuccessful campaign for the state's Fifth Congressional District seat. After the loss he established a legal practice in Ames, but he remained interested in politics. In 1974 he launched another bid for the Fifth Congressional District seat, and this time he defeated the Republican incumbent.

Harkin spent the next ten years in the U.S. House of Representatives, winning re-election four times in that span. In 1984 he successfully ran for the U.S. Senate, and he has been re-elected four times since then. During his years in the Senate, Harkin has garnered a reputation as one of Washington's most outspoken liberals, and as a leading policymaker on agriculture, education, and health care issues. He is perhaps best known, however, as an advocate for people with disabilities. In 1990, Harkin—who at the time was chairman of the Senate Subcommittee on Disability Policy—played a pivotal role in shepherding the landmark Americans with Disabilities Act (ADA) into law. Harkin was immensely proud of this legislation, which he has described as the Emancipation Proclamation for people with disabilities in the United States.

In addition to the ADA, Harkin has helped craft or pass numerous other disability-related pieces of legislation over the years, including the Developmental Disabilities Assistance and Bill of Rights Act of 1987, the Protection and Advocacy for Mentally Ill Individuals Amendments Act of 1988, the ADA Amendments Act of 2008, the Wellstone Mental Health Parity Act of 2008, and the Christopher and Dana Reeve Act of 2009. He is also a steadfast supporter of embryonic stem cell research.

Further Reading

McCrone, W. P. (1990, April). Senator Tom Harkin: Reflections on disability policy. *Journal of Rehabilitation, 56*(2), 8–10.

Tom Harkin: Iowa's senator (n.d.). Retrieved from http://harkin.senate.gov

Ted Henter (1950–)

Pioneering developer of screen reading software
for persons with visual impairments

Ted Henter was born in 1950 in the Panama Canal Zone, where his parents had also been raised. The only child of a father who worked as an engineer and a mother who worked as an office secretary and administrator, Henter attended primary school in the zone before earning a bachelor's degree in mechanical engineering from the University of Florida in 1974.

Henter's first dream was to carve out a career as a motorcycle road racer, and by 1978 he was ranked eighth on the global racing circuit. That year, however, he was blinded in an automobile accident in England. The accident derailed his career in motorcycle racing, but Henter recalls that "I got over feeling sorry for myself in about ten minutes." After weighing his options, Henter decided to shift to a career in computer programming. Henter took a number of computer courses at the University of South Florida, and by 1981 he was helping develop first-generation "talking" computers for people with vision impairments.

In 1985 Henter took his entrepreneurial and competitive instincts to the next level by establishing his own computer software business. Two years later, he and Bill Joyce founded Henter-Joyce and unveiled JAWS (Job Access With Speech), a revolutionary advancement in screen reading for computers. This screen reader software, which Henter toiled on for years with single-minded determination, translated text to speech so people who are blind or visually impaired can use a computer. JAWS was originally a DOS-based program, but by 1995 Henter-Joyce had developed a Windows version of the synthetic software package as well. JAWS thus became the most widely used screen reading software in the world by the late 1990s, and it had not relinquished this position a decade later.

In 2000 Henter-Joyce merged with two other assistive technology companies to form Freedom Scientific, which remains one of the titans of the AT industry. Henter serves as an advisor to the company, and he retains a seat on its board of directors. He has received numerous awards and honors for his contributions to assistive technology in general and his development of JAWS in particular, including special awards from the Smithsonian National Museum and the Association for Computing Machinery's Special Interest Group on Computer Human Interaction (SIGCHI).

In addition to his AT work, Henter is well known for his wide-ranging outdoor and sports interests. He has been a regular participant in a wide range of international races in such disciplines as canoe racing, martial arts, water skiing, and snow skiing.

Further Reading

Candela, T. (2004). Legends and pioneers of blindness assistive technology: Interview with Ted Henter. Retrieved from http://www.afb.org/Section.asp?SectionID=4&TopicID=456&SubTopicID=240&DocumentID=5497

Potok, A. (2002). *A matter of dignity: Changing the world of the disabled.* New York, NY: Random House.

Richard Hoover (1915–1986)

Educator who popularized the use of the long cane for people with blindness

Richard Edwin Hoover was born on January 19, 1915, in Wilkinsburg, Pennsylvania, a suburb of Pittsburgh. He obtained a bachelor of science degree from Pennsylvania State College (now Pennsylvania State University) in 1935 and earned his M.D. in ophthalmology from Johns Hopkins School of Medicine in 1950 with post-graduate work at Johns Hopkins Wilmer Institute.

Hoover's career as an educator began in 1936, when he took a teaching position at the Maryland School for the Blind. He taught mathematics and physical education and established a strong wrestling program at the school. When America entered World War II Hoover joined the U.S. Army. He was assigned to Valley Forge Army Hospital, where his duties centered on the care and rehabilitation of soldiers who had been blinded. Hoover's experiences at the Maryland School for the Blind and Valley Forge led him to develop a lightweight long cane for use by people with blindness and other severe sight impairments. Prior to this time, canes used by blind people were short tools made out of wood. Hoover conceived of a longer cane made out of lightweight materials. He combined this simple but elegant design with an "arcing" technique of deployment—one in which users could detect obstacles, changes in height, and other terrain features by swinging the tip of the cane side-to-side at ground level. Hoover also instituted a popular training program for use of the cane, which came into wide use during the late 1940s and 1950s.

After World War II concluded, Hoover returned to school, earning his ophthalmology degree from Johns Hopkins. He subsequently became an assistant professor of ophthalmology at Johns Hopkins Hospital and served on the staff of several hospitals in the Baltimore area—including a stint as chief of ophthalmology at Presbyterian Charity Hospital (where he started a residency program in 1959), which eventually became part of the Greater Baltimore Medical Center. Hoover remained with the program until his retirement in 1985.

Hoover served during his long career as a board director, consultant, or member to many notable public and private organizations concerned with issues related to blindness and disability. He also authored many scholarly papers on ophthalmology and blindness. Hoover received many honors and awards during his lifetime, including the Louis Braille Award from the Philadelphia Association for the Blind (1962), the Migel Medal from the American Foundation for the Blind (1970), and the Louis Braille Award from the Center for the Blind in Pennsylvania (1970). Hoover died on July 7, 1986.

Further Reading

American Printing House for the Blind (2011). Hall of fame: Richard Hoover. Retrieved from http://www.aph.org/hall_fame/bios/hoover.html
Welch, R. B. (1986). Richard Edwin Hoover, MD. *Transactions of the American Ophthalmological Society, 84,* 10–11.

Dean Kamen (1951–)

*Entrepreneur and inventor of a wide range
of medical products and assistive technology tools*

Dean Kamen was born on April 5, 1951, in Rockville Centre, New York. Even as a youth, he exhibited enormous intellectual curiosity, entrepreneurial zeal, and inventiveness. As a teenager, he became so adept at building sophisticated sound-and-light systems for concerts and other programs that his clients came to include Hayden Planetarium, the Four Seasons, the Museum of the City of New York, and the organizers of the Times Square New Year's Eve celebrations. After graduating from high school he attended Worcester Polytechnic Institute in Massachusetts. He spent more time on his personal engineering projects than schoolwork, however, and after five years WPI administrators ended his enrollment there.

As it turned out, Kamen's dismissal from WPI simply gave him more time to focus on his zeal for inventing. His first major breakthrough was a portable infusion pump with the capacity to deliver drugs to patients outside the hospital setting. In 1976 Kamen formed his first company, AutoSyringe Inc., to manufacture and market the pumps, which were especially useful to people with diabetic conditions.

In 1982 Kamen sold AutoSyringe to Baxter Healthcare Corporation. He then used the proceeds to renovate large sections of downtown Manchester and establish a new medical device company, called DEKA Research & Development. Under Kamen's visionary leadership, DEKA quickly became a prominent developer of new medical tools and devices for corporate clients in the health care industry. Triumphs in DEKA's early years ranged from revolutionary peritoneal dialysis systems to improvements in prosthetic limb technology.

In the 1990s Kamen shifted his attention to mobility devices, and by 2001 he had unveiled both the iBOT, a six-wheeled wheelchair capable of climbing stairs and navigating over rough terrain, and the Segway PT, a two-wheeled, self-balancing, electric-powered scooter. Sales and public acceptance of the Segway have not met Kamen's expectations, although the iBOT has been lauded for dramatically improving the lives of people with mobility problems in the United States and overseas. Unfortunately, after the iBOT was sold to Johnson and Johnson Corporation, production was halted in the mid-2000s. In recent years, Kamen's conviction that technology and science can solve pressing global problems has also led him to work on technological systems and innovations capable of addressing longstanding (and worsening) problems in developing nations, such as shortages of safe drinking water and environmentally sustainable energy.

In addition to DEKA, Kamen is devoted to the nonprofit organization FIRST (For Inspiration and Recognition of Science and Technology), which he founded in 1989. FIRST provides millions of dollars in scholarship funds on an annual basis to students interested in pursuing careers in science and technology and sponsors annual competitions in robotics and other technology areas.

Kamen has received many honors and awards over the years for his inventions. In 2000 he was awarded the National Medal of Technology in recognition for his role in advancing medical care for people with disabilities and other medical conditions. In 2002 he received the prestigious Lemelson-MIT Prize, and he was inducted into the National Inventors Hall of Fame in 2005.

Further Reading

Harris, M. (2009, July 22). Segway inventor on future technology—And why vide-
ogames aren't it. *Guardian* (UK). Retrieved from http://www.guardian.co
.uk/technology/2009/jul/22/dean-kamen-interview

Kemper, S. (2003). *Code name Ginger: The story behind Segway and Dean Kamen's
quest to invent a new world.* Boston, MA: Harvard Business Press.

Kirsner, S. (2009). Breakout artist. *Wired.* Retrieved from http://www.wired.com/
wired/archive/8.09/kamen_pr.html

Edward Kennedy (1932–2009)

American politician and supporter of disability rights legislation

Edward M. "Ted" Kennedy was born on February 22, 1932, in Boston, Massachusetts. The son of Joseph Patrick Kennedy, a businessperson and diplomat, and Rose (Fitzgerald) Kennedy, he hailed from a powerful political family. He graduated from Harvard University in 1956 and attended the International Law School in The Hague, the Netherlands, in 1958 before attaining his law degree from the University of Virginia the following year. He married Virginia Joan Bennet on November 29, 1958, and the couple raised three children before divorcing in 1981. Kennedy married Victoria Reggie in 1992.

Ted Kennedy was thrust into politics at an early age, helping manage his brother John F. Kennedy's senatorial and presidential campaigns in the late 1950s and early 1960s. After a brief tenure as the district attorney of Suffolk County in Massachusetts, he was elected to the U.S. Senate in November 1962. He would spend the next 47 years in Congress, becoming one of the nation's most powerful senators. He was also viewed as a viable presidential candidate, but his chances of gaining the White House were harmed by the Chappaquiddick scandal of 1969, when he was involved in an automobile accident that claimed the life of a female passenger in his car. Kennedy ended up entering just one presidential campaign, unsuccessfully seeking the Democratic nomination in 1980.

During his senatorial career, Kennedy was especially effective in championing legislation to benefit Americans with disabilities. His actions were partly inspired by his experiences with family members: his sister Rosemary was institutionalized for most of her life; his son Edward had his leg amputated during childhood; and another son, Patrick, was diagnosed with bipolar disorder. A supporter of the civil rights bills that became law in the 1960s, Kennedy later worked to broaden the scope of those protections to encompass citizens with disabilities and played a central role in passing laws that helped achieve important objectives of the disability rights movement.

Kennedy's early accomplishments included cosponsoring the Education for All Handicapped Children Act in 1975, which mandated that free and appropriate public education (FAPE) be made available to all children with disabilities. The following decade, he championed the Fair Housing Act Amendments of 1988, which extended the provisions of the 1968 housing legislation to apply to people with disabilities. In one of the crowning achievements of his career, Kennedy guided the landmark Americans with Disabilities Act through the Senate in 1990, and his leadership helped bring about overwhelming support for the bill in that chamber.

A series of other disability-related bills became law with Kennedy's assistance. These included the Family and Medical Leave Act (1993), which provided more options for caregivers; the Help America Vote Act (2002), which required equal access for disabled voters at polling places; the Assistive Technology Act (1988–2004), which supported state efforts to promote the development and use of assistive technology to improve the lives of people with disabilities; and the Family Opportunity Act (2006), which made Medicaid coverage available to a greater number of families with disabled children. During his final year in Congress, the senator helped win passage of the Genetic Information Nondiscrimination Act to prevent health care providers and employers from using an individual's genetic information in making employment and health coverage decisions.

In addition to these successes, Kennedy sought comprehensive health care reform for more than four decades, though he did not live to see that goal realized. He was diagnosed with brain cancer in 2008 and passed away on August 25, 2009, in Hyannis Port, Massachusetts.

Further Reading

Hersh, B. (2010). *Edward Kennedy: An intimate biography*. Berkeley, CA: Counterpoint.

Kennedy, E. (2009, July 18). The cause of my life. *Newsweek*. Retrieved from http://www.newsweek.com/2009/07/17/the-cause-of-my-life.html

A lifetime of service: Ensuring disabled Americans can live productive lives. (2009). Retrieved from http://tedkennedy.org/service/item/disability

Thomas King

*Speech-language pathologist who emphasizes
the "human factor" in assistive technology*

Wisconsin native Thomas Wayne King received his bachelor's degree from the University of Wisconsin-Madison, master's degrees from both the University of Wisconsin-Eau Claire and University of Wisconsin-Superior, and a doctoral degree from Clayton University. King then embarked on a long and distinguished career in the areas of assistive technology and augmentative communication. In his capacity as a certified speech-language pathologist and licensed and certified special educator and administrator, King worked and taught in a wide range of schools, clinics, universities, and private practice settings over more than three decades. Most notably, he worked for many years as the clinical supervisor of the Augmentative and Alternative Communication (AAC) and Assistive Technology (AT) Clinic at the University of Wisconsin-Eau Claire. He also founded and helped organize the annual Wisconsin Conference on AAC and AT and was elected first state president of the Wisconsin Society for Augmentative and Alternative Communication. King also collaborated with his wife, Dr. Debra King, to co-found Morse 2000 Worldwide Outreach, a collaborative outreach program in assistive technology.

King is the author of a number of academic and popular works on various disability and aging issues. His professional texts include *Modern Morse Code in Rehabilitation and Education: New Applications in Assistive Technology* (2000) and *Assistive Technology: Essential Human Factors* (1998). The latter work is particularly well known in the rehabilitation field for its emphasis on "human factors" when evaluating the effectiveness of assistive technology. According to King, people with special needs (and family members and other care providers) must be able to interact effectively and comfortably with assistive technology tools for them to be effective. In 2005 King retired from the University of Wisconsin-Eau Claire as professor emeritus of communication disorders.

Further Reading

King, T. (1998). *Assistive technology: Essential human factors.* Boston, MA: Allyn & Bacon.

Ray Kurzweil (1948–)

Author, futurist, and inventor whose inventions include an optical character-recognition machine for people with blindness

Ray Kurzweil was born on February 12, 1948, and grew up in the Queens borough of New York City. Kurzweil exhibited a passion for computer science and technology at an early age. In high school he created a sophisticated pattern-recognition software program that enabled him to create songs based on the styles of classical composers. The invention earned him a 1965 appearance on the television program *I've Got a Secret* and first prize at the 1965 International Science Fair. Three years later, while enrolled at Massachusetts Institute of Technology (MIT), Kurzweil devised a computer program that used various criteria to match high school students with colleges and universities. In 1970 he graduated from MIT with bachelor's degrees in both computer science and literature.

In 1974 Kurzweil founded Kurzweil Computer Products as a vehicle for pursuing various invention ideas, including a machine outfitted with optical character recognition (OCR) technology capable of identifying printed or typed documents regardless of printing quality or font style. The inventor then combined this "omni-font" (any font) OCR with a flatbed scanner and a text-to-speech synthesizer to create a pioneering print-to-speech reading machine for people who are blind. The Kurzweil Reading Machine was formally unveiled in January 1976, and it quickly became an essential assistive technology tool for many people with blindness and other visual impairments. In 1980 Kurzweil sold his company to Xerox, though he remained a consultant for the company for another 15 years.

Kurzweil's reputation as a modern-day Thomas Edison was further enhanced with a succession of new inventions during the 1980s and 1990s. A friendship with musician Stevie Wonder led Kurzweil to develop computerized music synthesizer programs capable of creating sounds that faithfully copy a wide range of acoustic instruments. These inventions were made available to the public through Kurzweil Music Systems, which was founded in 1982 (Kurzweil sold this company in 1990). Another company founded by Kurzweil in 1982—Kurzweil Applied Intelligence (KAI)—became a world leader in speech recognition technology. In 1996 Kurzweil launched Kurzweil Educational Systems, which quickly became a major player in the print-to-speech reading technology field.

In addition to his many inventions, Kurzweil has attracted considerable attention as a futurist. Several of his books, including *The Age of Intelligent Machines* (1990), *The Age of Spiritual Machines* (1998), *Fantastic Voyage: Live Long Enough to Live Forever* (2004), *The Singularity Is Near* (2005), and *Transcend: Nine Steps to Living Well Forever* (2009) have been bestsellers. He also maintains a Web site, KurzweilAI.net, that is immensely popular with readers interested in assistive technology, futurism, computers, and health and longevity.

Kurzweil has received numerous awards and honors over the course of his career. Honors of particular distinction include the 1994 Dickson Prize in Science, the 1998 MIT Inventor of the Year Prize, the 1999 National Medal of Technology, and the 2001 Lemelson-MIT Prize for a lifetime of developing assistive technology for people with disabilities. In 2002 Kurzweil was inducted into the National Inventors Hall of Fame for his invention of the Kurzweil Reading Machine.

Further Reading

A biography of Ray Kurzweil (n.d.). Retrieved from http://www.kurzweiltech .com/raybio.html

Castoro, R. (2009, April). Ray Kurzweil: That singularity guy. *Vice Magazine*. Retrieved from http://www.viceland.com/int/v16n4/htdocs/ray-kur zweil-800.php?page=1

Kurzweil, R. (2005). *The Singularity is near: When humans transcend biology.* New York, NY: Viking.

Ray Kurzweil: Inventor, author, futurist (n.d.). Retrieved from http://bigthink .com/raykurzweil

John Linvill (1919–2011)

American engineer, professor, and inventor of the Optacon

John Grimes Linvill was born on August 8, 1919 in Kansas City, Missouri. He attended William Jewell College in Liberty, Missouri, where he earned a bachelor of arts degree in mathematics in 1941. He then attended the prestigious Massachusetts Institute of Technology, earning a bachelor's degree in 1943, a master's degree in 1945, and a doctoral degree in 1949, all in electrical engineering.

Linvill spent two years at MIT as an assistant professor before moving to Bell Laboratories in 1951, where he focused on researching transistor circuits. His reputation as a proven teacher and outstanding researcher quickly spread. In 1954 he accepted an invitation from Stanford University to join the school's engineering faculty. He subsequently helped create Stanford's first transistor laboratory and played an important role in creating a circuit design and fabrication curriculum that would establish Stanford as a major supplier of engineers to the newly emerging computer industry in nearby Silicon Valley. He served as chair of the Department of Electrical Engineering from 1964 to 1980, and from 1972 to 1980 he also acted as dean of Stanford's School of Engineering.

Linvill is best known in the disability community for his invention of a reading machine called the Optacon, which he patented in 1966. The Optacon was a small, handheld camera that "translated" ordinary printed material onto a fingertip-sized tactile display that could be felt and interpreted by blind readers. The Optacon gave people with visual impairments far greater access to the written word. Linvill's invention of the device was inspired by his daughter Candy, who was blind. She illustrated the utility of her father's invention by using the Optacon while earning a doctorate in clinical psychology.

In 1970 Linvill co-founded Telesensory Systems Inc. to manufacture the Optacon. He received several awards in recognition of the invention, including the John G. McAulay Award from the American Association of Workers for the Blind in 1979, the John Scott Award in 1980, and the Louis Braille Prize in 1984. Meanwhile, he remained a prominent voice in the field of electrical engineering. He provided leadership and expertise as a member of the board of several Silicon Valley corporations and as a member of technical committees for the National Research Council, NASA, and the Institute of Electrical and Electronics Engineers. He was named a fellow of the Institute of Electrical and Electronics Engineers in 1960, and he was elected to the National Academy of Engineering in 1971 and the American Academy of Arts and Sciences in 1974. Linvill also was awarded the American Electronics Association's Medal of Achievement in 1983. Linville retired from Stanford as professor emeritus, and he died on February 19, 2011.

Further Reading

Myers, Andrew (2011, March 10). Stanford engineering professor and inventor, John G. Linvill, dies at 91. *Stanford Report*. Retrieved from http://news.stanford.edu/news/2011/march/john-linvill-obit-031011.html

Engineering memory of the month: The Optacon (June 2010). Retrieved from http://engineering/Stanford.edu/about/memories/06_2010_optacon.html

James C. Marsters (1924–2009)

Co-inventor of the text telephone system (TTY)

James Carlyle Marsters was born on April 5, 1924, in Norwich, New York. The son of a business executive and a nurse, Marsters lost his hearing when he was three months old after a bout with scarlet fever. He graduated from New York City's Wright Oral School for the Deaf in 1943 and earned a bachelor's degree in chemistry from Union College in Schenectady, New York, in 1947. He then gained admittance to the New York University School of Dentistry, albeit with a warning from administrators that the school would make no special provisions for him. Undaunted, Marsters excelled in his studies and graduated in 1952. Two years later he earned a master's degree in orthodontics at the University of Southern California (USC).

In 1954 Marsters opened an orthodontics practice in Pasadena that he maintained until his retirement in 1990. It is widely believed that in doing so, he became the first deaf orthodontist in the United States. He also served as a lecturer and clinical instructor in orthodontics for many years at USC. His wife, Alice, also worked in the Los Angeles area as a director at the John Tracy Clinic, which provides a wide range of services to the families of children with hearing loss.

Marsters is best known for his role in developing the text telephone system (TTY) that allows people with hearing impairments to communicate with each other by telephone from home without assistance. In 1964 he collaborated with two other men who were deaf, physicist Robert Weitbrecht and engineer Andrew Saks, in creating the first teletypewriter for use by deaf people. Their invention converted typed messages into audio tones that could be transported along standard telephone lines and converted back to message form. The machine, which Marsters promoted tirelessly, was described by scholar Harry G. Lange as a "technological declaration of independence for deaf people" that opened up new vistas of social and career opportunities for people with hearing impairments. Acceptance of the TTY modem technology developed by Marsters and his cohorts was slow in coming, in part because of resistance from telephone companies, but by the mid-1980s more than 180,000 TTY lines had been installed across the United States. Today, people who are deaf and hard of hearing are much less reliant on TTY systems for long-distance communication because they can utilize next-generation technology, such as instant messaging and e-mail.

Marsters retired from his orthodontics practice in 1990. That same year he received the AG Bell Association's highest award, "Honors of the Association," for his "extreme dedication to and sustained efforts to the betterment of the lives of people with hearing loss." Marsters died on July 28, 2009, in Oakland, California.

Further Reading

Lang, H. G. (2000). *A phone of our own: The deaf insurrection against Ma Bell.* Washington, DC: Gallaudet University Press.

Shapiro, T. R. (2009, August 28). James C. Marsters, 85; dentist co-created phone system for deaf. *Washington Post.* Retrieved from http://www.washington post.com/wp-dyn/content/article/2009/08/27/AR2009082703954.htm

Colin McLaurin (1922–1997)

Prosthetics designer and rehabilitation engineer

Colin McLaurin was born in Canada in 1922. As a young man he pursued an education in aeronautical engineering, and he served as a pilot in the Royal Canadian Air Force during World War II. After the war, though, his interests shifted to rehabilitation engineering. In 1949 he joined Sunnybrook Hospital in Toronto, a facility of the Canadian Department of Veterans Affairs. Over the next several years he joined with such researchers as James Foort and Fred Hampton to design new artificial hands and prostheses for military veterans.

The most momentous of their designs was a high-level prosthesis that featured an unlocked hip joint placed anterior to the acetabulum. This design, which McLaurin unveiled in 1954, positioned the center of gravity behind the mechanical hip joint and anterior to the knee joint during weight bearing, thus preventing the prosthesis from collapsing at the knee and hip. This sophisticated design (dubbed the Canadian Hip Disarticulation prosthesis) was widely recognized in the field of rehabilitation technology as a revolutionary breakthrough. Other advances made by McLaurin and his colleagues at Sunnybrook included the popularization of plastic laminate reinforcement for wooden prostheses and design of the Canadian Plastic Symes Prosthesis.

In 1957 McLaurin and Hampton accepted an offer to lead a new Northwestern University research program in Chicago. As the first director of the Prosthetic Research Center (now the Prosthetics Research Laboratory),

McLaurin played a vital role in guiding research and development work on prostheses. He also collaborated with George T. Aitken to develop the Michigan Feeder Arm, an electric, kinematically coupled artificial limb that could be utilized for daily activities by children born without arms.

In 1963 McLaurin moved to the Ontario Crippled Children's Center (now the Bloorview MacMillan Centre) in Toronto, where he served as that institution's first director of rehabilitation engineering. Over the next 14 years, McLaurin played a leading role in designing a multitude of prosthetics devices and rehabilitation aids, from advanced electric arms and mobility equipment to devices for grasping and using everyday household and office items. In addition, he helped establish a range of clinical services relating to prosthetics and orthotics at the center.

Another important contribution to the field of rehabilitation engineering was his chairmanship (from 1969 to 1975) of the Committee on Prosthetics Research and Development (CPRD) of NAS/NRC (National Academies of Science/National Research Council); during his tenure the CPRD formally endorsed increased funding and development of assistive technology centers. Moreover, CPRD during this time brought together leading clinicians and engineering researchers who formalized, justified, and documented the concept of rehabilitation engineering. McLaurin's clear vision of rehabilitation engineering—and his ability to articulate that vision to engineers, clinicians, and physicians—was pivotal throughout this period of growth.

In 1976 McLaurin took the helm at the University of Virginia's new Rehabilitation Engineering Center on Wheelchair Design and Development in Charlottesville, Virginia. As director of the center, he helped engineer many important and lasting improvements in wheelchair design. McLaurin also helped develop a master's program in rehabilitation engineering at the university. Finally, he played important parts in the founding of both the International Society for Prosthetics and Orthotics in 1972 and the Rehabilitation Engineering and Assistive Technology Society of North America (RESNA) in 1979. He also served as RESNA's second president. McLaurin died on August 5, 1997, at the age of 75.

Further Reading

Childress, D. S. (1998). A tribute to Colin A. McLaurin, 1922–1997. *Journal of Rehabilitation Research and Development, 35*(1), vii-x.

Harry J. Murphy

Director of the Center on Disabilities
at Cal State Northridge from 1983 to 2000

Harry J. Murphy began his college education at Philadelphia's Temple University, where he earned a bachelor's degree in education. Armed with a scholarship from the Office of Vocational Rehabilitation, he moved on to California State University, Northridge (CSUN), where he received a master's degree in leadership. Murphy then enrolled at the University of Southern California, where he earned his doctorate in educational psychology and administration.

Murphy's professional life began in Camden, New Jersey, where he worked briefly as a high school English teacher. He then accepted a teaching position at the Pennsylvania School for the Deaf in Philadelphia. After earning his master's degree from CSUN, Murphy took a research position at the John Tracy Clinic in Los Angeles, then served as principal of the Southwest School for the Deaf in Lawndale, California.

In 1972 Murphy began a nearly three-decade professional affiliation with CSUN when he accepted an assistant director position at CSUN's National Center on Deafness. He later became a professor of educational administration at the center.

In 1983 CSUN administrators approved the foundation of a new Center on Disabilities, which was dedicated to working to provide persons with disabilities all the training and research tools and assistive technologies they need for full inclusion in society. Murphy was the founding director of the center, and under his stewardship it became a national leader in disability research and assistive technology.

In 1985 the CSUN Center on Disabilities hosted the first International Conference on Technology and Persons with Disabilities. This conference, organized and conducted by Murphy and his staff, is now the longest-running and largest annual university-sponsored conference on technology and persons with disabilities. It serves as a major training venue for professionals around the world involved in the field of disability and assistive technology. The conference now typically attracts about 5,000 participants on an annual basis and includes presenters and exhibitors from all around the world.

Murphy retired in March 2000, but he remains actively involved in technology and disability issues. He has been formally recognized by the

National Council on Disability for his "outstanding leadership and services in the use of technology for people with disabilities," and in 2010 he was a recipient of the Roland Wagner Award from the International Conference on Computers Helping People with Special Needs (ICCHP).

Further Reading

Center on Disabilities, California State University at Northridge. Retrieved from http://www.csun.edu/cod/index.php
Kendrick, D. (2000, May). Dr. Harry Murphy: A man of vision. *AccessWorld, 1*(3). Retrieved from http://www.afb.org/afbpress/pub.asp?DocID=AW010302

James R. Reswick

Founding president of the Rehabilitation Engineering Society of North America (RESNA)

James Reswick's long and distinguished career began with faculty appointments at Case Western Reserve University, the Massachusetts Institute of Technology (MIT), and the University of Southern California (USC), where he directed one of the nation's first rehabilitation engineering research centers (RERCs) at USC-Rancho Los Amigos Hospital in Downey, California. Reswick also worked as a research scientist at the National Institute of Handicapped Research (NIHR), now known as the National Institute on Disability and Rehabilitation Research, and as director of the Rehabilitation Research and Development Evaluation Unit at the Veteran's Administration Medical Center in Washington, D.C., and Baltimore. In March 1988 Reswick was named associate director for research sciences of the National Institute on Disability and Rehabilitation Research. He served as acting director of the institute for two years.

Reswick made many contributions to the fields of assistive technology and rehabilitation engineering during his career, but he remains best known as one of the founders of the Rehabilitation Engineering Society of North America-RESNA (now known as the Rehabilitation Engineering and Assistive Technology Society of North America-RESNA). In August 1979 Reswick joined with fellow rehabilitation engineers Douglas Hobson, Colin McLaurin, Anthony Staros, and Joseph Traub to create the organization, which they envisioned as an interdisciplinary society that would bring science, engineering, and technology resources together to meet the needs of individuals with disabilities. Reswick was elected as RESNA's first president, and he remained a guiding voice within the organization for many years.

Since its founding, RESNA has carried out a wide array of programs related to rehabilitation engineering and assistive technology, including providing core technical assistance to numerous state and federal assistive technology initiatives; developing wheelchair testing standards; creating culturally sensitive training materials for assistive technology; and developing a certification program for professionals working as assistive technology service providers.

Reswick has retired, but he maintains a consulting and engineering design practice in the field of assistive technology for persons with disabilities. He is a member of the Institute of Medicine of the National Academy of Sciences and of the National Academy of Engineering. In addition, he is a fellow of the Institute of Electrical and Electronic Engineers and RESNA and an associate member of the American Academy of Orthopaedic Surgeons.

Further Reading

Hobson, D. A. (1996, December). RESNA: Yesterday, today, and tomorrow. *Assistive Technology: The Official Journal of RESNA, 8*(2), 131–143.

RESNA history (n.d.). Retrieved from http://www.resna.org/aboutUs/about Resna/about-resna-history.dot

Harry F. Rizer (1954–)

*Leading engineer and administrator
in the field of assistive technology*

Maryland native Harry F. "Bud" Rizer first made his mark in the field of assistive technology in the early 1980s. From 1982 to 1994 he served as technology resources office director for the Maryland State Department of Education's Division of Rehabilitation Services, Maryland Rehabilitation Center. For much of this same period he also was a part-time member of the faculty at the Johns Hopkins University School of Continuing Studies. In 1987 he received the Humanitarian Award from the National Rehabilitation Association. He earned his doctorate in special education and rehabilitation technology from Johns Hopkins in 1990.

In 1994 Rizer founded the T.K. Martin Center for Technology and Disability at Mississippi State University in Starkville. As the center's first director, he helped guide it to a position of national prominence in the field of rehabilitation technology after its formal opening in 1996. In mid-2000 he accepted the directorship of the renowned Center on Disabilities at California State University, Northridge (CSUN), which is dedicated to finding and disseminating electronics, computers, and other assistive technologies to students and other people with disabilities so as to enhance their participation in and access to the wider community.

Rizer worked at CSUN until 2005, when he accepted the position of executive director/chief executive officer at the National Cristina Foundation, an international not-for-profit organization based in Greenwich, Connecticut, that recycles computers and other donated technology for use by people with disabilities. The foundation's clientele includes charitable organizations, schools, and public agencies in all 50 states, Canada, and overseas.

In addition to his administrative work, Rizer has worked as a peer proposal reviewer for several federal agencies, consulted on assistive technology issues in China, Taiwan, and South Korea, and authored or co-authored a number of publications on disabilities and assistive technology.

Further Reading

Geuder, M. (1998, Spring). It's do-able: Technology comes to the aid of those with disabilities in state-of-the-art center. *Mississippi State Alumnus*. Retrieved from http://www.msstate.edu/web/alumnus/spring.98/08martin.htm

Green, C. (2010, February 5). National Cristina Foundation—Connecting used technology to worthy recipients. *Blue Planet Green Living*. Retrieved from http://www.blueplanetgreenliving.com/tag/national-cristina-foundation

Marcia Scherer

President and director of the
Institute for Matching Person and Technology

Marcia J. Scherer is known for her efforts to incorporate the needs of the whole person in assistive technology assessment and intervention. Scherer's research on the impact of assistive technologies on daily activities and societal involvement—and the measurement strategies she has devised for assessing those outcomes—has made her a luminary in the AT field.

When Scherer first attended college at Syracuse University, she intended to pursue a career in journalism. After earning a bachelor's degree in journalism in 1970, however, she shifted her course of study. In 1977 she earned a master's degree in rehabilitation and counseling from the University of Buffalo, and in 1986 she earned a master's degree in rehabilitation counseling and Ph.D. in family and work life studies from the University of Rochester.

Scherer secured her first professional position in 1985, when she took an assistant professorship with the National Technical Institute for the Deaf/Rochester Institute of Technology. She spent the next eleven years there, earning a promotion to associate professor in the spring of 1986. Later that same year, Scherer began a three-year stint as a senior research associate at the Department of Occupational Therapy's Center for Assistive Technology. In 1997 she also became an adjunct professor of physical medicine and rehabilitation at the University of Rochester's School of Medicine and Dentistry, a position she continued to hold through 2011. She also became editor of *Disability and Rehabilitation: Assistive Technology*, the official journal of the International Rehabilitation Medicine Association, in 2006.

Scherer is best known for her stewardship of the Institute for Matching Person and Technology, which she founded in 1997. The institute, which Scherer serves as both president and director, emphasizes the effective utilization of empirical measures and tools to facilitate the effective matching of individuals with disabilities with available assistive technologies.

Scherer has received numerous awards and honors in the fields of rehabilitation engineering and assistive technology, and she is a fellow of the American Psychological Association. Scherer has also served on the editorial board of several respected professional journals, and she has written or co-written a number of important books in the AT field, including *Living in the State of Stuck* (2005) and *Assistive technology in the Workplace* (2007).

Further Reading

Scherer, M. J. (2002, January). The importance of assistive technology outcomes. Retrieved from http://www.e-bility.com/articles/at.php

Scherer, M. J. (2004). *Connecting to learn: Educational and assistive technologies for people with disabilities.* Washington, DC: American Psychological Association (APA) Books.

Scherer, M. J. (2005). *Living in the state of stuck: How technology impacts the lives of people with disabilities.* Cambridge, MA: Brookline.

Kate Seelman (1938–)

American academic focusing on rehabilitation technology to advance independence in people with disabilities

Katherine D. Seelman was born on May 26, 1938. After receiving her bachelor's degree in history and political science from Hunter College in 1964, she pursued graduate studies at New York University, earning her master's degree in public policy in 1970 and her doctoral degree in science, technology, and public policy in 1982.

Seelman began her career as a community organizer in the 1960s, working in New York City and Little Rock, Arkansas. In 1986 Seelman, who is hard of hearing, became the director of public education for the Massachusetts Commission for the Deaf and Hard of Hearing. In 1989 she became a research specialist for the National Council on Disability, and in 1993 she was named the director of program development for the Administration of Developmental Disabilities, part of the U.S. Department of Health and Human Services. The following year she joined the National Institute on Disability and Rehabilitation Research, where she served as director until 2001.

In 2001 Seelman joined the faculty of the University of Pittsburgh, where she is associate dean and professor of rehabilitation science and technology at the School of Health and Rehabilitation Sciences, which is part of the Quality of Life Technology Center, a National Science Foundation Engineering Research Center run jointly by the University of Pittsburgh and Carnegie Mellon University. She also serves as an adjunct professor at Xian Jiaton University in China.

Seelman's research focuses on the development of science, technology, and public policy programs to create supports needed by people with disabilities and older adults to attain independence and community integration. She has shared her research as a representative of the United States in several international venues, including Japan and China, and also organized and directed a panel of disability specialists at the 2000 Rehabilitation International Meeting in Rio de Janeiro. Seelman also served on the international World Health Organization editorial committee, which released the first world report on disability in 2011.

Seelman has published many professional papers and books in the area of health and technology for persons with disabilities and aging adults. She is a contributor to *Handbook of Smart Technology for Aging* and *Disability and Independence: Computing and Engineering Design and Application*, and co-editor of *Handbook of Disability Studies*. She is the recipient of many awards, including the Gold Key Award from the American Congress of Rehabilitation Medicine, the Distinguished Public Service Award from the American Academy of Physical Medicine and Rehabilitation, and a Switzer Fellowship.

Further Reading

Linkov, F., LaPorte, R., & Seelman, K. D. (2010). Cancer, disability and public health service providers: Better education through informatics and the Supercourse. *International Journal of Public Policy, 6*(3/4), 247–257.

Seelman, K. D., Collins, D. M., Bharucha, J. A., & Osborn, J. (2007). Giving meaning to quality of life through technology: Cutting-edge research on aging-in place technologies at Carnegie Mellon University/University of Pittsburgh. *Nursing Homes, 56*(10), 40–42.

Anthony Staros (1923–2008)

Longtime director of the VA Prosthetics Research Center and leading figure in the formation of RESNA and the International Society for Prosthetics and Orthotics

Anthony "Tony" Staros was born on July 17, 1923. He earned a master's degree in engineering at Massachusetts Institute of Technology (MIT), then interrupted his schooling to serve as a first lieutenant in the U.S. Marine Corps' Infantry and Aviation Logistics section during World War II. After the war, Staros went back to school (attending Cornell University, Stanford University, and Hofstra University) and obtained a second master's degree in engineering. He then became a licensed professional engineer in the state of New York.

In 1951 Staros joined the Department of Veterans Affairs (VA), which dramatically increased its involvement in prosthetics research and other types of assistive technology after the 1954 passage of the Vocational Rehabilitation Act. In 1956 Staros established the VA Prosthetics Center (VAPC) in New York City. This facility, which combined traditional clinical offerings with research and development initiatives in physical therapy, prosthetics/orthotics, facial restoration, wheelchair standards and design, orthopedic medicine, and other assistive technologies, was the first of its kind in the United States. Under Staros's guiding hand, VAPC developed numerous innovative rehabilitation practices and assistive/augmentative devices for disabled veterans over the next few decades. During this period, in fact, the center became the nation's leading provider of custom-engineered prosthetics, orthotics, orthopedic shoes, and other assistive technologies to veterans with physical disabilities. In 1964 Staros founded a publication, *The Bulletin of Prosthetics Research,* to publicize the mission and successes of VAPC. This journal eventually expanded into the *Journal of Rehabilitation Research and Development,* which is a leading voice in the realm of assistive technology.

In addition to his work with VAPC, Staros was one of the five founding members of the Rehabilitation Engineering Society of North America (RESNA) in 1979. He also played a leading role in the 1970 establishment of International Society for Prosthetics and Orthotics (ISPO) in Copenhagen, Denmark. Staros served as president of ISPO's second world congress and as its third president. After retiring he served as senior program consultant for World Rehabilitation Fund initiatives around the world, including Lebanon, Dominican Republic, Haiti, Vietnam, and Uganda. He also continued to make regular contributions to scholarly journals dedicated to the study of orthotics, prosthetics, and other assistive technologies. Staros died in New York City on July 20, 2008.

Further Reading

McAleer, J. (2008). In memoriam: Anthony Staros. *Journal of Rehabilitation Research & Development, 45*(9), xv.

Reswick, J. B. (2002, November/December). How and when did the rehabilitation engineering center program come into being? *Journal of Rehabilitation Research and Development, 39*(6), 11–16.

Staros, A. (1981). Rehabilitation engineering and prosthetics/orthotics. *Clinical Prosthetics & Orthotics, 5*(4), 1–3.

Joe Traub (1928?–1990)

Leading administrator of federal and private rehabilitation engineering programs in the post-World War II era

Joseph Traub was born in the late 1920s in Fort Wayne, Indiana. He was born with missing bones in his fingers and without a large bone in his right leg. His right leg was amputated when he was a toddler. Traub originally intended to pursue a career in teaching, but after three years of study at the University of Indiana, he decided to enroll in the Institute of

Rehabilitation Medicine in New York City. It was there that he received his early grounding in prosthetics, orthotics, and other rehabilitation engineering work. He then spent five years at the University of Buffalo as the school's director of prosthetics and orthotics.

In 1956 Traub moved to California, where he became a researcher and instructor in rehabilitation engineering at the University of California at Los Angeles (UCLA). In 1963 he went to the University of Washington, where he designed curricula for prosthetics and orthotics instruction. One year later, however, he joined the Veterans Administration (VA; now the Department of Veterans Affairs). This federal agency had vaulted to the forefront of assistive technology research in the late 1950s and early 1960s, in large part because of a productive collaboration with the National Academy of Sciences (NAS) and the U.S. Department of Health, Education, and Welfare (HEW). Together, they created the Committee on Prosthetics Research and Development (CPRD), which modernized assistive technology tools and rehabilitation research across the country.

In 1967 Traub moved over to HEW, where he oversaw funding of a multitude of research programs created by CPRD and other organizations to improve the efficacy of wheelchairs, reading machines, prosthetics, orthotics, and other assistive technologies. Over the next several years, Traub also worked with Anthony Staros (of the VA), A. Bennett Wilson Jr. (of the National Research Council), and Jim Garrett (of the Rehabilitation Services Administration) to develop an influential model for national rehabilitation engineering centers (RECs).

The rehabilitation engineering center concept was first formally defined at a meeting held by the CPRD at Annapolis, Maryland, in September 1970. Representatives of the federal government and persons deeply involved in the field of rehabilitation research, education, and patient service, formulated guidelines for the establishment of rehabilitation engineering centers of excellence. Traub and Garrett then led an intensive lobbying effort that resulted in a provision in the landmark Rehabilitation Act of 1973 ensuring that one quarter of research funding under the act would go to RECs.

As funding for REC programs increased, Traub and other leaders in the assistive technology and rehabilitation engineering fields agreed that information exchange between the centers would be essential to maximizing research and rehabilitation results. Traub thus became one of the five founding members of the Rehabilitation Engineering Society of North America (RESNA) in 1979. Traub died of cancer in Alexandria, Virginia, on October 13, 1990.

Further Reading

Reswick, J. B. (2002, November/December). How and when did the rehabilitation engineering center program come into being? *Journal of Rehabilitation Research and Development, 39*(6), 11–16.

Taylor, C. (1990, October 25). Joseph Traub, pioneered techniques, equipment for fellow disabled people. *Seattle Times.* Retrieved from http://community .seattletimes.nwsource.com/archive/?date=19901025&slug=1100472

Pellegrino Turrl

Italian inventor credited with creating the first functional typewriter

Very little is known about Pellegrino Turri, but in 1808 the Italian inventor made an important contribution to the development of assistive technology by creating what is thought to be the first working typewriter. Although the details are murky and, for the most part, lost to history, the apparent motivation behind his invention makes this a fascinating story. Turri was in love with the Countess Fantoni da Fivizzono, but there were two problems: both Turri and the Countess were married to others, and the Countess was going blind. Her visual impairment made it impossible for them to continue their written correspondence in a discreet fashion, as the Countess did not want to involve a third party for dictation and risk compromising their relationship. Turri solved this problem by building a machine that the Countess could use on her own to write love letters to him. Turri never patented his machine, perhaps because he needed to keep its existence a secret, or perhaps because he did not fully realize its importance. Although the Countess did not save the machine, a few of the letters that she wrote on it are preserved in the town of Reggio, Italy, thus proving its existence and utility.

Apart from Turri's little-known breakthrough, the historical development of the modern typewriter was a very slow process. Henry Mill of England was granted a patent in 1714 for creating a machine for printing letters, but he was never able to build a working version. Ralph Wedgwood, also of England, worked on similar technology around the same time as Turri and created an apparatus for that purpose that used an early version of carbon paper. Turri's typewriter also used carbon paper, so some historians credit him with inventing it as well. There is no known connection between Wedgwood and Turri, however, and it is impossible to know for certain who created it first.

Turri did not survive long enough to realize the far-reaching implications of his invention. A commercially successful version of the typewriter with the modern QWERTY keyboard would not come until nearly 70 years later, developed by American inventor and newspaper publisher Christopher Sholes. There is no doubt, however, that the development of the typewriter—and its 20th century descendant, the personal computer—was a milestone in the history of communication, not only as an assistive technology for people who are blind, but as a tremendous time-saver for all people. The fact that Turri was motivated by his love for a woman who was blind inspired the creation of a novel, *The Blind Contessa's New Machine* (2010) by Carey Wallace.

Further Reading

Adler, Michael H. (1973). *The writing machine*. London: Allen & Unwin.
Polt, Richard. (n.d.). The classic typewriter page. *A brief history of typewriters*. Retrieved from http://staff.xu.edu/polt/typewriters/tw-history.html

Gregg Vanderheiden

Pioneer in the field of augmentative communication and director of the Trace Center

Gregg C. Vanderheiden's academic career unfolded at the University of Wisconsin in Madison, where he received a bachelor's degree in electrical engineering (1972), a master's degree in biomedical engineering (1974), and a Ph.D. in technology in communication rehabilitation and child development (1984). Simultaneous with these studies, Vanderheiden made his mark as a pioneer in the fields of assistive technology and augmentative communication (the latter a term he himself coined and popularized). In 1971 he joined with several colleagues and students to found the Student Cerebral Palsy Communication Instrumentation Group at the University of Wisconsin. Vanderheiden served as founding director of the group, which eventually became the internationally known Trace Research & Development Center. He also became a professor of industrial and biomedical engineering at the University of Wisconsin-Madison.

Under Vanderheiden's guidance, the Trace Center became an important voice on technology and communication issues for people with disabilities during the 1970s and 1980s. Many of the accessibility features for people with disabilities that were built into Macintosh, Windows, and Linux computer operating systems during this era were developed by Vanderheiden and the Trace Center in 1984, when the center served as a coordinator for the national Industry-Government Initiative on Computer Accessibility.

Vanderheiden built on this success in the late 1980s and 1990s, when the Trace Center partnered with the computer industry to integrate disability access features into their mass-market products. This initiative succeeded in incorporating disability access features into virtually all computer operating systems—a state of affairs that remains in place today.

In 2008 Vanderheiden co-founded Raising the Floor (RtF), an organization dedicated to ensuring universal access to the latest communication and computer technology. He has also been a leading voice in National and Global Public Inclusive Infrastructures—campaigns to build full accessibility and usability functions into the Internet's infrastructure. A past president of RENSA, Vanderheiden also directs the NIDRR Rehabilitation Engineering Research Center (RERC) on Universal Interfaces and Information Technology Access, and co-directs the RERC on Telecommunications Access (joint with Gallaudet University) in addition to his continued work as director of the Trace Center.

Vanderheiden has received numerous honors and awards during his career, including the ACM Social Impact Award from the Human-Computer Interaction Community (2005), the Ron Mace Designing for the Twenty-First Century Award (2000), the Access Award from the American Foundation for the Blind (1991), and the Isabelle and Leonard H. Goldenson Award for Outstanding Research in Medicine and Technology (1978).

Further Reading

Pfaff, K. (1995, January). Ensuring access. *TeamRehab Report*, 30–31.

Vanderheiden, G. C. (2006). Design for people with functional limitations. In G. Salvendy (Ed.), *Handbook of human factors and ergonomics* (pp. 1387–1417). New York, NY: Wiley.

A. Bennett Wilson, Jr.

Mechanical engineer and longtime director of the
Committee on Prosthetic Research and Development (CPRD)

A. Bennett Wilson, Jr. was one of the leading originators of the generalized rehabilitation engineering movement in the United States. As executive director of the Committee on Prosthetic Research and Development (CPRD), he joined with other influential figures in assistive technology including Joseph Traub, Colin McLaurin, and James Reswick to obtain major governmental support and funding for rehabilitation engineering centers (RECs), which during the 1970s and 1980s became a central hub of rehabilitation and assistive technology for people with disabilities.

This shift began in the mid-1950s, when the U.S. Department of Health, Education, and Welfare (HEW) used funds generated by the 1954 Vocational Rehabilitation Act to establish new prosthetic and orthotic research and development programs. Rehabilitation studies and initiatives in the United States were initially carried out under separate schemes for civilians and military veterans. During the 1960s, however, researchers on both sides of this divide increasingly recognized the importance and wisdom of sharing information. Leading administrators subsequently established a Committee on Prosthetics Research and Development (CPRD) within the National Academy of Science's National Research Council to help guide the expansion of rehabilitation engineering centers, assistive technology research, and other elements of the rehabilitation engineering movement.

As the longtime director of CPRD, Wilson worked closely with officials in the Department of Veterans Affairs and other agencies. Under his leadership, the CPRD became well-known for its ability to bring together most of the leaders and workers in the field of rehabilitation engineering through active subcommittees, ad hoc committees, and workshops. These meetings, in turn, encouraged the development of new research priorities and the careful evaluation of new devices and systems.

In addition to his efforts to disseminate scholarly information about new assistive technology innovations and amputation techniques, Wilson also played a notable role in establishing modern medical nomenclature regarding prosthetics and amputations. He died in July 2001.

Further Reading

Reswick, J. B. (2002, November/December). How and when did the rehabilitation engineering center program come into being? *Journal of Rehabilitation Research and Development, 39*(6), 11–16.

Wilson, A. B., Jr. (1998). *Primer on limb prosthetics.* Springfield, IL: Charles C. Thomas.

Wilson, A. B., Jr. (1971). Limb prosthetics today. *Artificial Limbs, 7*(2), 1–42.

Joy Zabala

Educator who emphasizes the use of assistive technology to extend learning opportunities to people with disabilities

Joy Smiley Zabala received her bachelor of arts degree in education from the University of Florida and her master's degree in education from

Florida Atlantic University. She then earned a doctorate in education from the University of Kentucky. In addition, she is credentialed as an assistive technology practitioner by the Rehabilitation Engineering and Assistive Technology Society of North America-RESNA.

For much of her professional life, Zabala has worked in general and special education environments to provide training to teachers, students, families, education agencies, organizations, and companies in the use of assistive technology (AT). A frequent speaker on all aspects of assistive technology, from selection and implementation of AT options to evaluations of their effectiveness, Zabala also developed the SETT Framework—Student-centered, Environmentally useful, Tasks-focused Tool systems. She describes SETT as a methodology for students, parents, and teachers to use when assessing the capacity of AT options to promote student achievement.

Zabala is a founding member of the QIAT (Quality Indicators for Assistive Technology) Community and a former president of the Technology and Media Division (TAM) of the Council for Exceptional Children. From 2007 to 2009 she served as project manager of the AIM Consortium, a collaborative effort between multiple state agencies and the Center for Applied Special Technology (CAST) to extend specialized educational materials to students with special instructional needs. In her capacity as director of technical assistance at CAST, Zabala also has been heavily involved in universal design issues in education settings. In addition, she directs the technical assistance efforts of the National Center on Accessible Instructional Materials and serves as the evaluator of the NIMAS (National Instructional Materials Accessibility Standard) Development Center, which was created to provide students with traditional print disabilities with access to educational sources in other formats, including Braille, digital text, and audio. She also serves on the advisory boards of the Family Center for Technology and Disability and Bookshare.

Further Reading

Zabala, J. S. (2005). Using the SETT Framework to level the learning field for students with disabilities. Retrieved from http://www.joyzabala.com/uploads/Zabala_SETT_Leveling_the_Learning_Field.pdf

Zabala, J. S. (n.d.). About Joy. http://joyzabala.com/About.html

Five

Annotated Data, Statistics, Tables, and Graphs

Cathy Bodine, Lorrie Harkness, and Maureen Melonis

A number of important factors provided impetus for acceleration in the development of the field of assistive technology (AT). These factors included returning soldiers requiring ongoing rehabilitation following World War II, growing numbers of individuals with disabilities surviving infancy, and improvements in overall medical care for those who sustained traumatic injuries. Positive changes in how society was beginning to perceive those with disabilities also played a significant role, leading to legislative initiatives supporting the inclusion of persons with disabilities into mainstream life activities.

Advancements in technology and personal computers also played a critical role in the forward momentum of the field. Technology offers a means for individuals with disabilities to be independent and achieve their personal goals. With technical advancements and a growing recognition of the need for trained professionals, organizations such as the Rehabilitation Engineering Society of North America (RESNA) and the International Society of Augmentative and Alternative Communication

(ISAAC) formed in the late 1970s and early 1980s. Professional journals dedicated to AT also began to emerge at this time.

This chapter provides a synthesis of key work to date in the field and includes relevant data, statistics, and graphs on important findings. The information has been organized by category to facilitate understanding. Because the field of AT draws upon research from many diverse fields—such as rehabilitation engineering, occupational, physical, and speech-language therapies, education, etc.—the information below is categorized by content areas. The first area is a general overview of disability prevalence. The next area includes age-based categories such as AT and Early Intervention, AT and Education, AT and Employment, AT and Veterans, and AT and Aging. These are followed by categories related to the field, including AT Funding (includes state financing) and AT Training. The next area includes AT for specific disability categories, such as Mobility and Movement, Communication, and Vision and Hearing. The final categories include Prevalence of AT Use, Public Access to AT (including computers, the Internet, equipment recycling programs, and device demonstrations), Barriers to AT and Social Participation, and finally AT Sales and Industry Data.

Disability

In understanding the application of assistive technology, it is paramount to first have a general understanding of the incidence of disability. The tables below provide general information on the incidence of disability in the United States taken from the U.S. Census Bureau. The Census Bureau conducts numerous studies of population and demographics. Three of those summaries are provided in this section.

Every ten years, surveys are distributed to all residents in the United States, and in 2000 the results indicated that almost 1 in 5 Americans had a disability (U.S. Census Bureau, 2002). Table 1 includes disability data by age group and gender.

The American Community Survey (ACS), an ongoing statistical survey conducted by the U.S. Census Bureau, gathers information previously collected every ten years to analyze demographic, housing, social, and economic trends. Rather than surveying the entire population, the ACS gathers data from a sample of residents, sending questionnaires to 3 million homes per year. Information is gathered from every state and Puerto Rico. This new data collection process was launched in 1995 and began producing test data in 2000, 2001, and 2002. The full program was implemented by 2010. In 2008, the estimated percentage of the overall

Table 1 Characteristics of the Civilian Noninstitutionalized Population by Age, Disability Status, and Type of Disability: 2000

Characteristic	Total		Male		Female	
	Number	Percent	Number	Percent	Number	Percent
Population 5 and older	257,167,527	100.0	124,636,825	100.0	132,530,702	100.0
With any disability	49,746,248	19.3	24,439,531	19.6	25,306,717	19.1
Population 5 to 15	45,133,667	100.0	23,125,324	100.0	22,008,343	100.0
With any disability	2,614,919	5.8	1,666,230	7.2	948,689	4.3
Sensory	442,894	1.0	242,705	1.0	200,188	0.9
Physical	455,461	1.0	251,852	1.1	203,609	0.9
Mental	2,078,502	4.6	1,387,393	6.0	691,109	3.1
Self-care	419,018	0.9	244,824	1.1	174,194	0.8
Population 16 to 64	178,687,234	100.0	87,570,583	100.0	91,116,651	100.0
With any disability	33,153,211	18.6	17,139,019	19.6	16,014,192	17.6
Sensory	4,123,902	2.3	2,388,121	2.7	1,735,781	1.9
Physical	11,150,365	6.2	5,279,731	6.0	5,870,634	6.4

(Continued)

Table 1 (Continued)

Characteristic	Total		Male		Female	
	Number	*Percent*	*Number*	*Percent*	*Number*	*Percent*
Mental	6,764,439	3.8	3,434,631	3.9	3,329,808	3.7
Self-care	3,149,875	1.8	1,463,184	1.7	1,686,691	1.9
Difficulty going outside the home	11,414,508	6.4	5,569,362	6.4	5,845,146	6.4
Employment disability	21,287,570	11.9	11,373,786	13.0	9,913,784	10.9
Population 65 and older	33,346,626	100.0	13,940,918	100.0	19,405,708	100.0
With any disability	13,978,118	41.9	5,634,282	40.4	8,343,836	43.0
Sensory	4,738,479	14.2	2,177,216	15.6	2,561,263	13.2
Physical	9,545,680	28.6	3,590,139	25.8	5,955,541	30.7
Mental	3,592,912	10.8	1,380,060	9.9	2,212,852	11.4
Self-care	3,183,840	9.5	1,044,910	7.5	2,138,930	11.0
Difficulty going outside the home	6,795,517	20.4	2,339,128	16.8	4,456,389	23.0

Source: U.S. Census Bureau, 2000 Census of Population and Housing, *Summary File 3: Technical Documentation,* 2002.

Note: For information on confidentiality protection, sampling error, nonsampling error, and definitions, see http://www.census.gov/prod/cen2000/doc/sf3.pdf.

Table 2   The Percentage of Noninstitutionalized Persons in the United States Who Reported a Disability: 2008

Location	Estimate (%)	90% MOE	Base Population	Sample Size
United States	12.1	± 0.05	299,852,800	2,949,415
Alabama	16.1	± 0.39	4,593,900	46,329
Alaska	12.0	± 0.84	680,700	6,256
Arizona	12.0	± 0.29	6,426,800	60,643
Arkansas	17.6	± 0.52	2,808,300	28,268
California	10.2	± 0.11	36,326,400	340,770
Colorado	9.4	± 0.30	4,880,400	48,105
Connecticut	10.4	± 0.38	3,446,700	34,133
Delaware	12.8	± 0.82	861,900	8,100
District of Columbia	10.9	± 0.93	583,900	5,412
Florida	12.8	± 0.18	18,057,000	181,737
Georgia	11.7	± 0.24	9,537,200	92,647
Hawaii	10.1	± 0.61	1,280,500	13,025
Idaho	12.0	± 0.61	1,503,600	15,280
Illinois	10.3	± 0.20	12,730,100	124,434
Indiana	12.7	± 0.30	6,276,700	64,676
Iowa	11.8	± 0.40	2,954,500	30,152
Kansas	12.3	± 0.45	2,757,100	27,676
Kentucky	17.0	± 0.42	4,207,100	42,383
Louisiana	14.9	± 0.39	4,329,400	41,648
Maine	15.7	± 0.73	1,302,900	12,401
Maryland	10.2	± 0.29	5,563,100	55,367

(Continued)

Table 2 (Continued)

Location	Estimate (%)	90% MOE	Base Population	Sample Size
Massachusetts	11.3	± 0.29	6,405,400	63,757
Michigan	13.2	± 0.25	9,873,000	98,707
Minnesota	9.5	± 0.30	5,154,700	52,173
Mississippi	16.7	± 0.50	2,882,700	28,390
Missouri	14.1	± 0.33	5,816,900	58,981
Montana	13.2	± 0.80	954,300	8,936
Nebraska	10.3	± 0.53	1,757,000	17,630
Nevada	10.1	± 0.43	2,578,000	25,475
New Hampshire	11.3	± 0.64	1,301,100	12,842
New Jersey	9.8	± 0.23	8,571,600	85,496
New Mexico	13.6	± 0.56	1,960,800	18,262
New York	11.2	± 0.16	19,239,200	183,849
North Carolina	13.0	± 0.26	9,107,700	91,104
North Dakota	10.9	± 0.90	630,900	6,520
Ohio	13.1	± 0.23	11,310,700	114,573
Oklahoma	16.5	± 0.45	3,573,500	35,612
Oregon	13.3	± 0.40	3,749,100	36,729
Pennsylvania	13.4	± 0.22	12,221,900	122,445
Rhode Island	12.7	± 0.75	1,037,000	9,999
South Carolina	13.9	± 0.38	4,413,200	44,296
South Dakota	11.0	± 0.81	788,300	7,856
Tennessee	14.8	± 0.33	6,129,100	61,904
Texas	11.6	± 0.15	23,942,300	229,787
Utah	8.9	± 0.40	2,715,800	26,502

Location	Estimate (%)	90% MOE	Base Population	Sample Size
Vermont	14.4	± 0.95	615,600	5,930
Virginia	10.7	± 0.26	7,660,300	77,182
Washington	12.0	± 0.29	6,492,100	64,623
West Virginia	19.2	± 0.63	1,790,000	17,779
Wisconsin	10.7	± 0.30	5,546,100	57,211
Wyoming	12.7	± 0.98	526,400	5,423
Puerto Rico	21.2	± 0.44	3,926,400	32,203

Source: Erickson, W., Lee, C., & von Schrader, S., *Disability statistics from the 2008 American Community Survey (ACS)*, Cornell University Rehabilitation Research and Training Center on Disability Demographics and Statistics (StatsRRTC), 2010.

population with a disability—regardless of sex, age, race, ethnicity, or education level—based on the sample for each state was 12.1% for the entire United States and Puerto Rico. The lowest estimate was 8.2% for Utah, and the highest 21.2% for Puerto Rico. The next-highest estimate was 19.2% for West Virginia.

Another tool for evaluating disability prevalence is the Current Population Survey (CPS). Also conducted by the Census Bureau, the CPS is focused on labor force statistics and gathers data from a representative sample of the total population living in residential homes. The information is used to evaluate employment levels and the economic status of households. Table 3 reflects the percentage of men and women, aged 18 to 64, who report a work limitation in the United States in five-year moving averages. The percent has remained below 8% from 1981 to 2007.

AT and Early Intervention

The 28th Annual Report to Congress in 2009 collected data on the number of infants and toddlers from birth to age 2 served under the Individuals with Disabilities Education Act (IDEA), Part C, who received AT devices or services (U.S. Department of Education, 2009). The numbers are based on reporting on Individualized Family Service Plans (IFSP). Part C of the Individuals with Disabilities Education Act (1997 amendments) mandates

Table 3   The Percent of Working Individuals Reporting a Work Limitation
Over Five-Year Spans

Year	Percent (%)	95% MOE	Average Sample Size
2003–2007	7.8	± 0.1	125,887
2002–2006	7.8	± 0.1	126,849
2001–2005	7.7	± 0.1	117,554
2000–2004	7.6	± 0.1	108,690
1999–2003	7.5	± 0.1	99,191
1998–2002	7.6	± 0.1	89,221
1997–2001	7.7	± 0.1	79,253
1996–2000	7.8	± 0.1	79,144
1995–1999	7.8	± 0.1	80,792
1994–1998	7.9	± 0.1	82,771
1993–1997	7.9	± 0.1	85,523
1992–1996	7.8	± 0.1	88,485
1991–1995	7.6	± 0.1	91,968
1990–1994	7.4	± 0.1	93,188
1989–1993	7.2	± 0.1	92,663
1988–1992	7.1	± 0.1	92,857
1987–1991	7.1	± 0.1	92,857
1986–1990	7.2	± 0.1	92,776
1985–1989	7.3	± 0.1	93,159
1984–1988	7.4	± 0.1	95,162
1983–1987	7.4	± 0.1	95,920
1982–1986	7.4	± 0.1	96,630
1981–1985	7.4	± 0.1	99,268

Source: Von Schrader, S., Erickson, W. A., & Lee, C. G., *Disability statistics from the Current Population Survey (CPS)*, 2010. Retrieved from http://www.disabilitystatistics.org.

AT be considered when planning and implementing IFSPs. A comprehensive multidisciplinary evaluation of each child's strengths and needs must identify resources appropriate to meet the needs of the child, including assistive technology. Statements about early invention services, including assistive technology devices and services and how they will be delivered, must be part of the Individual Family Service Plan (IFSP). Parental input is vital in the selection and implementation of assistive technology. Despite legal requirements and significant efforts to promote the use of AT for young children with disabilities, it is frequently omitted from family service plans and is underutilized by individuals with disabilities of all ages, particularly young children. Nationally, AT interventions are documented on only 3.1% of the IFSPs (U.S. Department of Education, 2009).

Table 4 Infants and Toddlers, Birth to Age 2, Who Received AT Under IDEA, Part C, by State, Fall 2003

State	AT Services/Devices	State	AT Services/Devices
Alabama	22	Idaho	33
Alaska	7	Illinois	795
Arizona	36	Indiana	1,073
Arkansas	7	Iowa	9
California	210	Kansas	263
Colorado	74	Kentucky	461
Connecticut	411	Louisiana	140
Delaware	6	Maine	118
District of Columbia	x	Maryland	197
Florida	60	Massachusetts	220
Georgia	444	Michigan	28
Hawaii	86	Minnesota	413

(Continued)

Table 4 (Continued)

State	AT Services/Devices	State	AT Services/Devices
Mississippi	x	South Dakota	41
Missouri	352	Tennessee	325
Montana	46	Texas	33
Nebraska	40	Utah	12
Nevada	63	Vermont	5
New Hampshire	14	Virginia	49
New Jersey	32	Washington	151
New Mexico	9	West Virginia	154
New York	522	Wisconsin	244
North Carolina	81	Wyoming	x
North Dakota	23	50 states and D.C.	8,091
Ohio	137	American Samoa	x
Oklahoma	547	Guam	x
Oregon	21	Northern Marianas	12
Pennsylvania	21	Puerto Rico	169
Rhode Island	48	Virgin Islands	266
South Carolina	7	U.S. and outlying areas	8,541

Source: Office of Special Education Programs, U.S. Department of Education, *Twenty-eighth Annual Report to Congress on the Implementation of the Individuals with Disabilities Education Act,* Table 6-6, Washington, DC, 2009.

The 28th Annual Report to Congress in 2009 also indicated the number of infants and toddlers receiving AT as categorized by race and ethnicity, as shown in Table 5.

Table 5   Infants and Toddlers, Birth to Age 2, Receiving AT Under IDEA, Part C, by Race and Ethnicity, 1998–2003

Infants and Toddlers Receiving AT						
Year	American Indian/ Alaska Native	Asian/ Pacific Islander	Black (Not Hispanic)	Hispanic	White (Not Hispanic)	Race/ Ethnicity Total
1998	52	169	1,079	1,193	4,518	7,011
1999	76	248	1,460	1,571	5,236	8,591
2000	106	176	1,009	1,632	6,045	8,968
2001	94	246	964	1,247	5,539	8,090
2002	110	303	1,065	1,087	5,981	8,546
2003	91	287	1,130	1,061	5,552	8,121

Source: Office of Special Education Programs, U.S. Department of Education, *Twenty-eighth Annual Report to Congress on the Implementation of the Individuals with Disabilities Education Act*, Table 6-12a, Washington, DC, 2009.

AT and Education

With the passage of such pivotal legislation as the Individuals with Disabilities Education Act (IDEA), Section 504 of the Rehabilitation Act of 1973, and the Education for All Handicapped Children Act (Public Law 94–142), the field of education has had a major impact on the field of AT and the AT industry. The essential elements of the law are threefold and intended to ensure (1) that AT is considered for all children who may benefit, (2) that an appropriate assessment is conducted, and (3) that AT devices and services are provided to those who are eligible. Nationally, every child with a disability who has an Individualized Educational Plan (IEP) must have documentation determining if the use of AT was considered. IDEA requires that teams determine if a child requires AT devices and services in order to receive a free appropriate public education (FAPE). The team must document the type of device and service on the child's IEP.

Below are figures indicating the number of students who receive AT through their IEP. Figure 1 indicates the percent of teachers using AT implementation plans. It is based on a survey of rural districts in

Figure 1   Percent of Teachers Using AT Implementation Plans

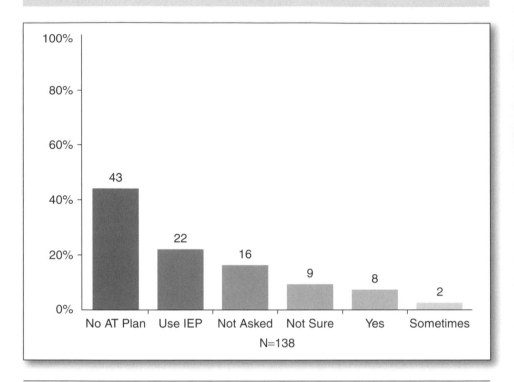

Source: Bausch, M. E., & Ault, M. J., *Nationwide use of assistive technology implementation plans,* National Assistive Technology Research Institute (NATRI), University of Kentucky, 2005.

ten participating states. It indicates that only 8% had an AT implementation plan in place for their students. Of the remaining 91% of teachers, 43% had no AT plan, 22% used the IEP plan, 16% were not asked, 9% were not sure, and 2% used a plan sometimes.

In addition to providing access to the general education curriculum, legislation requires the consideration of AT for access to testing. When President George W. Bush signed the No Child Left Behind Act into law in 2002, a national move toward standards-based education reform began. States were required to provide accommodations on testing for children with disabilities who needed them. Those accommodations include AT devices *and* services.

Table 6 is taken from the 2007 Annual Report on Participation and Accommodations alternate assessments of student performance in schools

Table 6   Equipment and Material Accommodations Allowed, State
Alternative Assessments

C2—Equipment and Material Accommodations			
Option	Allowed (A)	Allowed With Qualifications (A*)	Prohibited (P)
Magnification equipment	51	0	0
Amplification equipment	48	1	0
Light/acoustics	37	1	0
Calculator	12	41	1
Templates	41	0	1
Audio/video equipment	18	10	0
Noise buffer	35	1	0
Adaptive/ special furniture	32	1	0
Abacus	23	10	1
Manipulatives	14	10	2
Adapted writing tools	23	1	0
Slant board/wedge	9	1	0
Secure paper to work area	11	1	0
Visual organizers	21	1	0
Color overlay	20	0	0
Assistive technology	18	12	1
Special paper	22	1	0
Math tables/numberline	7	12	4
Dictionary/glossary	11	13	2
Thesaurus	0	6	2
Keyboard	10	0	0
Graphic organizers	10	2	0

Source: Altman, J., Thurlow, M., & Vang, M., *2007 Annual Report on Participation, Annual Performance Report: 2007–2008;* State Assessment Data, National Center on Educational Outcomes (NCEO), 2010.

Note: Twelve additional accommodations were added in 2007: Adapted Writing Tools, Slant Board/Wedge, Secure Paper to Work Area, Visual Organizers, Color Overlay, Assistive Technology, Special Paper, Math Tables/Number Line, Dictionary/Glossary, Thesaurus, Keyboard, and Graphic Organizers (Christensen, Lazarus, Crone, & Thurlow, 2008).

across the nation and in U.S. territories. Students who take the alternate assessment most often have disabilities, and some students who are not proficient in English are also eligible. Many of the accommodations allow the use of AT to take the test. The National Center on Educational Outcomes (NCEO) has led numerous assessment projects and conducted research on students with disabilities' participation and performance on statewide assessments since 1992 (Altman, Thurlow, & Vang, 2010). According to this data, the most common types of accommodations, equipment, or material provided are magnification and amplification equipment. It is interesting to note that AT is also listed as one of the categories. Table 6 shows the number of states and territories that provide specific accommodations. For example, the first accommodation is for magnification equipment. Fifty-one states/territories allow the accommodation, 0 states allow it with qualifications (designated A*), and 0 states prohibit it (P). This information demonstrates how many states/territories have an accommodation policy.

Access to AT is a challenge in many service delivery models. A study published in 2009 examined data from the 2001 U.S. National Survey of Children with Special Health Care Needs. The survey involved over 18,000 children from 0 to 17 years of age who required AT. Results found an estimated 49% of children with special health care needs required AT services such as vision or hearing aids, mobility and communication devices, and other medical equipment. The study examined met and unmet needs in AT, as well as whether those unmet needs were associated with having a quality medical home, access to therapy, and enrollment in early intervention or special education. Table 7 presents the findings.

Figure 2 presents a comparison of unmet versus met need for assistive devices by service categories among U.S. children with special health care needs, ages 0 to 17, needing all devices (Figure 2a) and needing only communication, hearing, or mobility devices (Figure 2b).

The National Assessment of Educational Progress (NAEP) measures national trends in student performance in mathematics, reading, and other academic subjects. The average 4th-grade NAEP mathematics score in 2009 was higher than the score in 1990, but unchanged from the score in 2007. The average 8th-grade mathematics score in 2009 was higher than the score in all previous assessment years and 2 points higher than the score in 2007. Figure 3 illustrates these trends. The average NAEP reading score at Grade 4 increased by 4 points, from 217 to 221

Table 7   Analysis of Unmet Needs for Assistive Technology Among U.S. Children Ages 0–17 With Special Health Care Needs

	Unmet need for all assistive devices, O.R. (95% C.I.)*		
	Quality medical home (n= 14,938)	Early intervention/ special education (n= 17,416)	Therapy services (n= 5026)
Services received			
Yes	–	–	–
No	3.27 (2.29-4.66)	0.86 (0.68-1.10)	3.52 (2.25-5.48)
Level of severity			
Mildly or not severe	–	–	
Moderately severe	1.34 (0.97-1.86)	1.47 (1.08-2.01)	1.32 (0.76-2.29)
Most severe	2.22 (1.57-3.15)	2.52 (1.80-3.53)	2.87 (1.72-4.78)
Gender			
Male	–	–	–
Female	1.15 (0.91-1.47)	1.16 (0.92-1.46)	0.98 (0.68-1.42)
Age			
< 3 years	–	–	–
3-5 years	0.99 (0.53-1.87)	1.31 (0.63-2.70)	1.47 (0.60-3.58)
6-11 years	1.79 (1.02-3.13)	2.21 (1.12-4.33)	1.67 (0.72-3.88)
12-17 years	2.10 (1.21-3.65)	2.64 (1.36-5.13)	2.28 (0.98-5.27)
Race			
Caucasian only	–	–	–
African-American only	1.24 (0.89-1.74)	1.32 (0.94-1.86)	1.16 (0.68-1.98)
Multiracial	2.13 (1.26-3.61)	2.44 (1.48-4.03)	3.41 (1.55-7.52)
Other	0.63 (0.37-1.08)	0.87 (0.49-1.54)	1.25 (0.67-2.33)
Hispanic			
Yes	–	–	–
No	0.71 (0.48-1.05)	0.70 (0.47-1.06)	0.79 (0.43-1.44)

(Continued)

Table 7 (Continued)

Family structure			
1 adult	–	–	–
2 adults	0.82 (0.57-1.16)	0.80 (0.57-1.14)	0.71 (0.44-1.15)
3 adults	0.93 (0.60-1.45)	0.92 (0.60-1.42)	0.61 (0.32-1.17)
4 or more	0.66 (0.38-1.16)	0.64 (0.37-1.10)	0.78 (0.36-1.70)
Family size			
1 child	–	–	–
2 children	0.73 (0.54-1.00)	0.76 (0.57-1.02)	0.88 (0.54-1.41)
3 children	0.88 (0.61-1.25)	0.80 (0.56-1.14)	1.20 (0.74-1.97)
4 or more	0.89 (0.61-1.31)	0.84 (0.58-1.23)	0.99 (0.57-1.73)
Poverty level			
≥400% FPL	–	–	–
200-399% FPL	1.12 (0.70-1.78)	1.27 (0.81-1.99)	1.02 (0.60-1.73)
<200% FPL	**2.40 (1.48-3.89)**	**2.53 (1.58-4.06)**	1.72 (0.99-2.98)
Maternal education			
4-year degree or more	–	–	–
Some secondary	0.88 (0.63-1.23)	0.90 (0.65-1.24)	0.76 (0.48-1.21)
High school graduate	**0.62 (0.44-0.87)**	**0.60 (0.43-0.84)**	**0.51 (0.32-0.82)**
Less than high school	**0.66 (0.44-0.99)**	**0.66 (0.44-0.98)**	**0.47 (0.25-0.86)**
Underinsurance			
Always covered and adequate	–	–	–
Always covered but inadequate	**2.49 (1.89-3.29)**	**2.88 (2.20-3.78)**	**1.73 (1.20-2.48)**
Intermittent coverage	**4.51 (2.94-6.92)**	**5.77 (3.77-8.85)**	**2.70 (1.23-5.92)**
No coverage in past year	**7.28 (4.82-10.98)**	**8.44 (5.62-12.67)**	**3.57 (1.72-7.41)**

Source: Benedict, R. E., & Baumgardner, A. M., A population approach to understanding children's access to assistive technology, Table 3, *Disability and Rehabilitation, 31*(7), 582–592, 2009. From 2001 to 2002 National Survey of Children with Special Health Care Needs.

Note: *Odds ratios in bold are significant at p = 0.05.

(on a scale of 0–500) between 1992 and 2009, but was unchanged from the average score in 2007. At Grade 8, the 2009 average reading score (264) was 4 points higher than the score in 1992 and 1 point higher than the average score in 2007. Although the data is not disaggregated, allowable testing accommodations appear to be having a positive impact on test scores.

Figure 2   Comparison of Unmet Versus Met Need for Assistive Devices Among U.S. Children Needing All Devices and Needing Only Communication, Hearing, or Mobility Devices

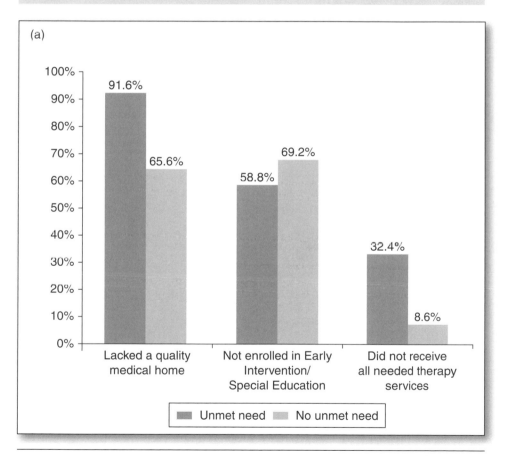

(Continued)

Figure 2 (Continued)

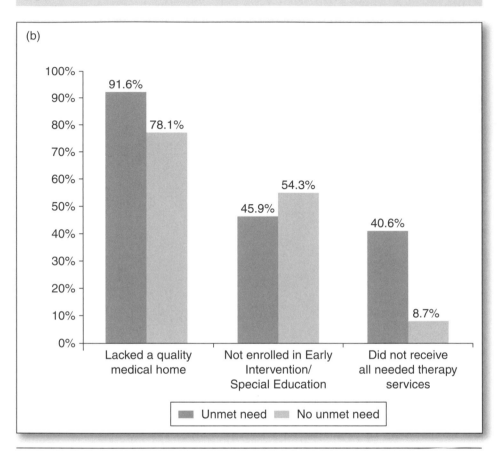

Source: Benedict, R. E., & Baumgardner, A. M., A population approach to understanding children's access to assistive technology, Table 3, *Disability and Rehabilitation, 31*(7), 582–592, 2009. From 2001 to 2002 National Survey of Children with Special Health Care Needs.

AT and Employment

Among working-age people, AT has the potential to promote personal independence and better work outcomes. According to a National Council on Disability study of people who received assistive technology, it had a significant positive impact on their lives. For example, 62% of working-age persons indicated that they were able to decrease their dependence on caregivers. More significantly, the report indicated that 58% were able to reduce their dependence on paid assistance, while 37% were able to

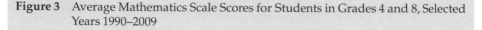

Figure 3   Average Mathematics Scale Scores for Students in Grades 4 and 8, Selected
Years 1990–2009

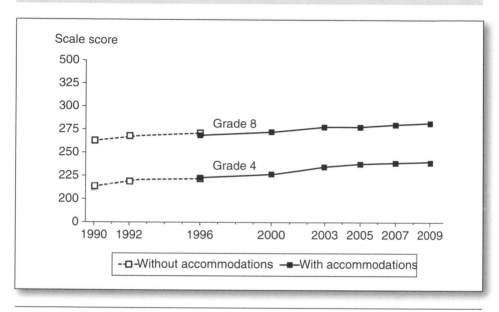

Source: U.S. Department of Education, National Center for Education Statistics, *National Assessment
of Educational Progress,* Figure 24-1, 2010. Retrieved from http://nces.ed.gov/programs/coe/
figures/figure-mat-1.asp.

Note: Data are available for 1990, 1992, 1996, 2000, 2003, 2005, 2007, and 2009. In early years of the
assessment, testing accommodations (e.g., extended time, small group testing) for children with disabilities and limited-English-proficient students were not permitted. In 1996, scores are shown for
the assessments with and without accommodations to show comparability across the assessments.

increase earnings. AT users also reported improvements in overall quality
of life. Ninety-two percent indicated that AT helped them to work faster or
better, while over 80% indicated AT enabled them to earn more money
(National Council on Disability, 1993).

Four-fifths (81%) of employers responding to a 1995 Harris poll said
that they had made accommodations for workers with disabilities, up
from half (51%) in 1986. But even if employers are making greater efforts to
provide job opportunities for people with disabilities, national surveys still
do not conclusively show increased levels of employment (Kaye, 1998). As
of 2012, the Office of Disability Employment Policy (ODEP) reports current
labor force participation as 20.7% for persons with disabilities and 70% for
persons without disabilities. The unemployment rate for persons with disabilities is 13.6%, and for persons without disabilities it is 8.4%. Figure 4
examines employment trends among people with disabilities.

Figure 4   Employment Trends Among People With Disabilities, 1990–1995

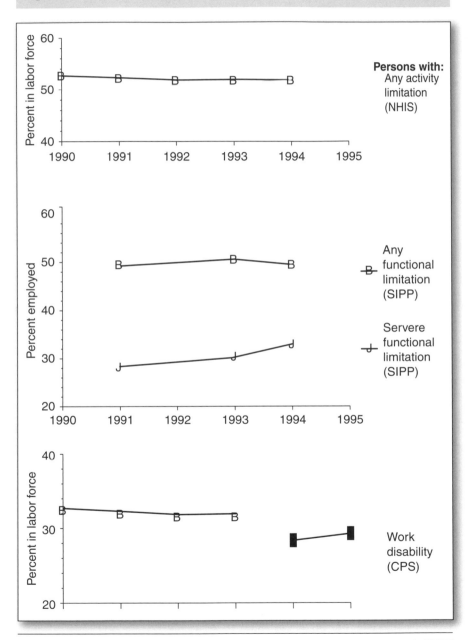

Source: Kaye, S., Is the status of people with disabilities improving?, Figure 1, UCSF Disability Statistics Center, 1998. Retrieved from http://dsc.ucsf.edu/figure.php?pub_id=7&section_id=1&figure_id=1.

State Vocational Rehabilitation (VR) programs evaluate clients to determine whether assistive technology can provide them with the tools they need to be successfully employed. Rehabilitation technology services is the term used in the VR program for the application of technology solutions to problems that individuals with disabilities face in their day-to-day functioning, including the use of assistive technology and assistive technology services. Table 8 shows the percentage of VR clients in the 50 United States and the District of Columbia who participated in these evaluations prior to exiting the system in 2009. The range of percentages among states ranged from 00.0% to 17.1%.

Table 9 shows, for those cases that closed into an employment setting having rehabilitation technology services, whether the setting was for competitive employment or not (Smith, Butterworth, Domin, & Hall, 2012). Employment categories include employment without supports in integrated settings; self-employment (except BEP); state agency-managed Business Enterprise Program (BEP); small businesses operated by individuals with significant disabilities under the State VR agency; homemaker; unpaid

Table 8   Provision of Rehabilitation Technology Services to VR Cases Closed

United States	No Service	Service	Total
	94.2%	5.8%	580,295

Table 9   Provision of Rehabilitation Technology by Work Setting in VR Cases Closed

Employment Without Supports—Integrated Setting	Self-Employment (Except BEP)	BEP	Homemaker	Unpaid Family Worker	Employment With Supports—Integrated Setting	Not Competitively Employed	Competitively Employed
13%	27%	80%	51%	18%	4%	30%	13%
1997	1070	147	2166	60	714	2608	21346

Source: Adapted from Smith, F. A., Butterworth, J., Domin, D., & Hall, A. C., Data Note: VR Outcome Trends and the Recent Decline in Employment for VR Customers with Intellectual Disabilities, *Data Note Series,* Institute for Community Inclusion, Paper 2, 2012. Retrieved from http://scholarworks.umb.edu/ici_datanote/2.

Note: Data covers United States and District of Columbia, 2009. Total number of closures into work settings: 23,954.

family worker (a person who works without pay on a family farm or in a family business); employment with supports in integrated setting. Competitive employment means work that is compensated at or above the minimum wage. An individual who is not competitively employed is one who is being compensated at less than minimum wage or is working as a homemaker or unpaid family worker. Overall, 13% of the closures received rehabilitation technology services.

AT and Veterans

Computer/Electronics Accommodations Program (CAP)

The Department of Defense's Computer/Electronic Accommodations Program (CAP) has provided assistive technology to military personnel and federal employees with disabilities since its authorization in 2001. Soon after the implementation of the CAP program, a pilot project emerged to assist wounded service members. The 2008 Annual Stakeholders Report indicates that over 10,000 requests for accommodations were filled in that year.

Figure 5 depicts the accommodations profile by disability type for 2008 and includes wounded service members. Figure 6 shows the

Figure 5 Accommodations Profile by Disability Type, Including Wounded Service Members, 2008

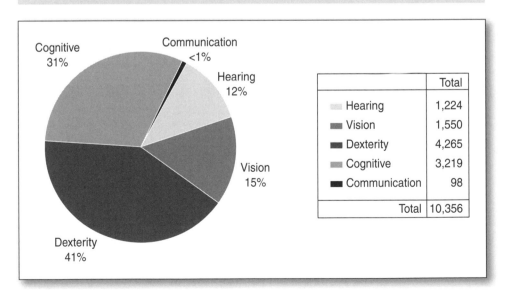

	Total
Hearing	1,224
Vision	1,550
Dexterity	4,265
Cognitive	3,219
Communication	98
Total	10,356

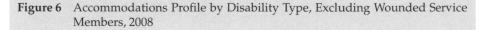

Figure 6   Accommodations Profile by Disability Type, Excluding Wounded Service
Members, 2008

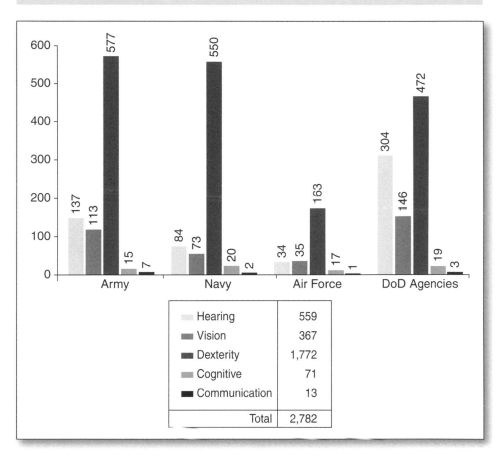

accommodations profile for the same year but excludes wounded service members. Figure 7 shows how the CAP program benefited wounded service members over five years, beginning in 2004.

Figure 8, the Wounded Service Members Profile for Fiscal Year 2008, shows that most of the accommodations provided by CAP were for members of the Army. Service members who are injured during active duty are provided the technology and related services that are needed for their rehabilitation and then allowed to keep the technology and continue any needed services when they separate from active duty free of charge.

Figure 7   Wounded Service Members Accommodations Profile, 2004–2008

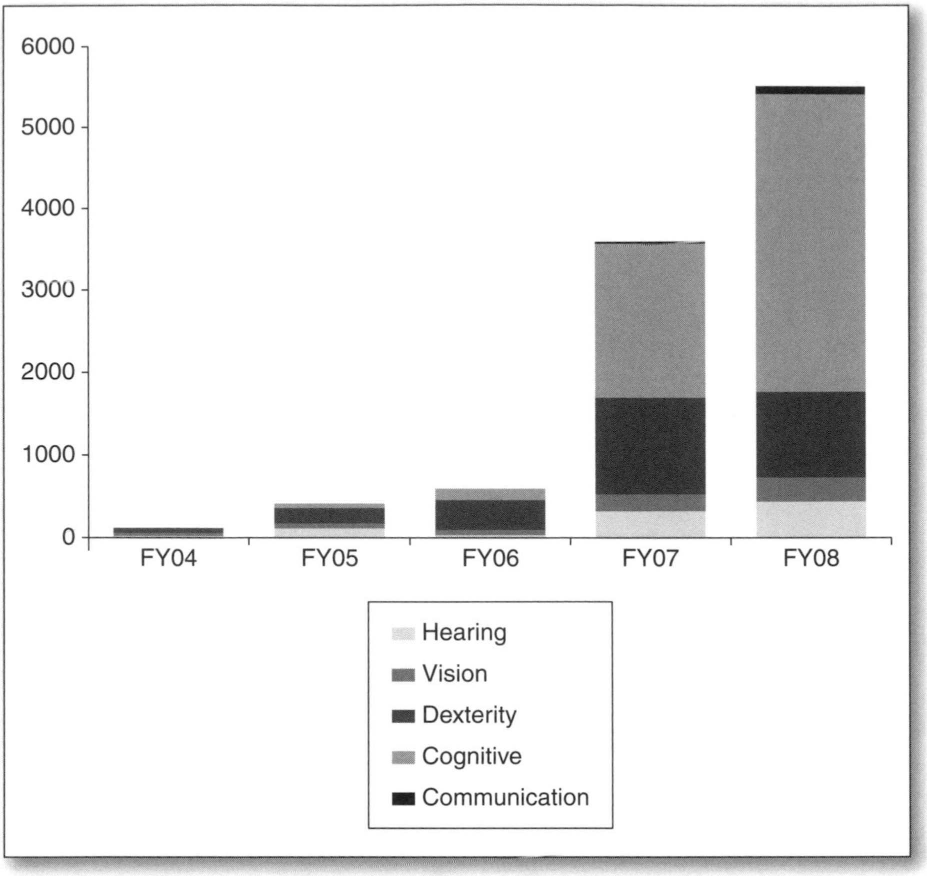

Source: U.S. Department of Defense, Office of the Assistant Secretary of Health Affairs, TRICARE Management Activity, *Real Solutions for Real Needs,* in *CAP Annual Stakeholders Report,* 2008.

AT and Aging

As demographic changes in the United States trend toward a greater aging population, the need for assistive technology increases. There is a clear correlation between the need for AT devices and services and aging. Research indicates that seniors use AT more than other groups (Mann, Goodall, Justiss, & Tomita, 2002; Mann, Hurren, Tomita, & Charvat, 1997), as shown in Figure 9. Assistive technology offers seniors a means to greater independence.

Figure 8 Wounded Service Members Profile, 2008

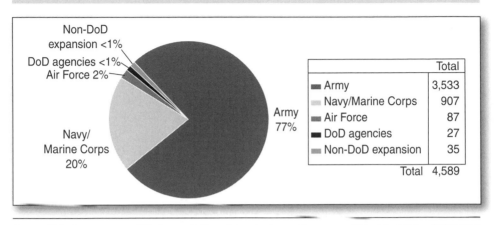

Source: U.S. Department of Defense, Office of the Assistant Secretary of Health Affairs, TRICARE Management Activity, *Real Solutions for Real Needs*, in *CAP Annual Stakeholders Report*, 2008.

Figure 9 Estimated Number of People Using AT and Home Access Features, by Age Group

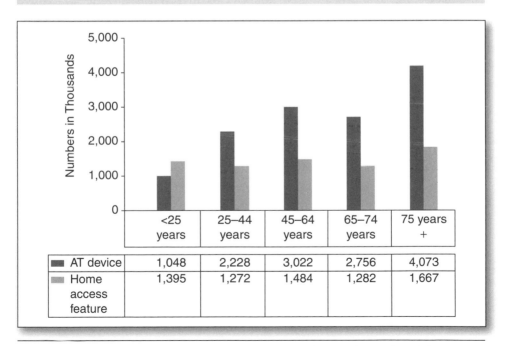

Source: LaPlante, M. P., Hendershot, G. E., & Moss, A. J., The prevalence of need for assistive technology devices and home accessibility features, *Technology and Disability, 6,* 17–28, 1997.

AT Funding

Assistive technology devices and services are funded by a number of private, state, and federal sources. Nationally, the Tech Act Programs focus on improving access to and acquisition of assistive technology through state-level activities and leadership. Formula grants administered by the U.S. Department of Education Rehabilitation Services Administration provide funding to each state and territory based on total population (U.S. Department of Education, 2006). Reauthorization of the Tech Act in 2004 required four state-level activities, including state financing, device reutilization, device loan, and device demonstration programs. In addition, state leadership activities included training, technical assistance, public awareness and information, coordination, and collaboration. Table 10 shows the funding by source for all states, as well as for states receiving other funding. Total Tech Act funding for 2009 was $25,660,000.

Funding of assistive technology can be provided through a number of public and private sources, including insurance, educational and vocational systems, state and local agencies, and out-of-pocket purchases. Table 11 indicates the breakdown of typical funding sources for AT devices and home modifications, and indicates whether they were paid for out of pocket, by third-party payors, or by a combination of both.

Table 10   Amount of Funding and Percentage of Total Funding, by Source, FY 2004

Funding Source	All States (n=54)		States Receiving Other Funding (n=33)	
	Amount	Percentage of Total	Amount	Percentage of Total
Title I	$20,035,863	52	$12,544,235	41
Other	$18,400,600	48	$18,400,600	59
Total	$38,436,463	100	$30,944,835	100

Source: LaPlante, M. P., Hendershot, G. E., & Moss, A. J., The prevalence of need for assistive technology devices and home accessibility features, *Technology and Disability, 6,* 17–28, 1997.

Table 11   Funding Sources for AT Devices and Home Modifications

	AT Devices	*Home Access Features*
Out of pocket	48.2%	77.5%
Third party	34%	15.2%
Combination	17.9%	7.3%

Source: LaPlante, M. P., Hendershot, G. E., & Moss, A. J., The prevalence of need for assistive technology devices and home accessibility features, *Technology and Disability, 6,* 17–28, 1997.

State financing activities, as part of the State Tech Act Programs, can assist individuals with disabilities in obtaining AT devices and services. These activities vary from state to state and may include financial loan programs as well as other activities to help individuals acquire AT. In the 2012 Tech Act report, 28 states reported having at least one financial loan program. Depending on the loan program, the major types of purchases were for vehicle modifications and transportation (74%). Most of the remaining funds (14%) were for hearing aids (U.S. Department of Education, 2009).

AT Training

Assistive technology without accompanying training is not assistive. National Tech Act data indicates that training is provided to professionals, individuals with disabilities, their family members, students, employers, and policymakers. The 2009 Tech Act report shows that 62,344 individuals participated in training that was offered. The participants profile appears in Figure 10.

The geographic representation of these participants was 68% metropolitan, 23% non-metropolitan, and 9% unknown. Training topics and percentage of participants were distributed as shown in Table 12.

In 2009, 218,000 individuals received information and assistance in response to inquiries about assistive technology. It was estimated that 18,202,731 people were reached with AT information through public-service announcements, Internet information, print materials, newsletters, listservs, exhibits, and other means.

Figure 10   Recipients of AT Training

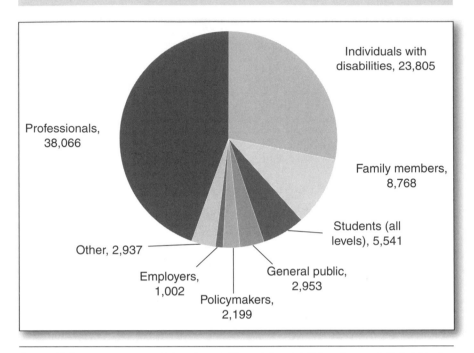

Source: U.S. Department of Education, Office of Special Education and Rehabilitative Services, Rehabilitation Services Administration, *Annual Report to Congress on the Assistive Technology Act of 1998 for Fiscal Years 2004 and 2005,* 2009. Retrieved from http://www2.ed .gov/about/reports/annual/rsa/atsg/2004/index.html.

Table 12   Percentage of Participants in AT Training by Topic

Topic	Percentage
AT products and services	47
AT funding/policy	7
IT/telecommunications access	7
Transition and AT	13
Combination	25

Source: U.S. Department of Education, Office of Special Education and Rehabilitative Services, Rehabilitation Services Administration, *Annual Report to Congress on the Assistive Technology Act of 1998 for Fiscal Years 2004 and 2005,* 2009. Retrieved from http://www2.ed.gov/about/reports/annual/rsa/atsg/2004/index.html.

Assistive Technology by Disability Categories

AbleData indicates that, as of 2010, there were almost 40,000 assistive technology product listings in 20 categories in their database of AT products. The AbleData AT product offerings included disability categories, such as Blind and Low Vision and Deaf and Hard of Hearing, as well as functional categories, such as Communication, Education, Housekeeping, Recreation, Safety and Security, and Transportation.

AT for Mobility and Movement

Assistive technology for mobility and movement includes devices designed to aid an individual with disabilities in moving his/her body within or between environments. It includes items such as wheelchairs, prosthetics, and walking aids. There has been a steady growth in demand for mobility devices, partly due to growth in the aging population, an increase in survival rates following trauma, along with improvements in the technology itself (LaPlante, Hendershot, & Moss, 1992). For example, the number of individuals using wheelchairs and walkers doubled from 1980 to 1990. In addition, use of crutches increased by 14% and use of canes increased by 53% in this same period. Since 1990, this steady growth has continued (Russell, Hendershot, LeClere, Howie, & Adler, 1997).

Data from the National Health Interview Survey (NHIS) conducted by the U.S. Census Bureau for the National Center for Health Statistics, part of the Centers for Disease Control and Prevention (CDC), indicate that use of mobility devices is rising. Over 6.8 million Americans living outside of institutions use AT for mobility assistance. Of this group, 1.7 million use wheelchairs or scooters. Ninety percent of these individuals use manual (versus power) wheelchairs or scooters. Regarding other types of mobility devices, such as canes, crutches, and walkers, use is at 6.1 million (see Table 13). The most common mobility devices are canes (used by 4.8 million Americans), walkers (1.8 million), and crutches (566,000).

For the 6.8 million Americans with mobility impairments living in their local communities, there are a number of differences as compared to their counterparts without disabilities. For example, they are more than 40 times more likely to need help with self-care activities. They are often combating secondary health conditions, including arthritis, stroke, or serious back problems. They may have other debilitating impairments or conditions, such as multiple sclerosis or spinal cord or other type of paralysis. The vast majority has lower socioeconomic status and many more hospitalizations than the general population.

Table 13   Number of Persons Using Assistive Technology Devices by Age of Person and Mobility Device: United States, 1994

	All ages	44 years and under	45–64 years	65 years and over
Mobility devices	Number in thousands			
Any mobility device	7,394	1,151	1,699	4,544
Crutch	575	227	188	160
Cane	4,762	434	1,116	3,212
Walker	1,799	109	295	1,395
Medical shoes	677	248	226	203
Wheelchair	1,564	335	365	863
Scooter	140	12	53	75

Source: U.S. Centers for Disease Control, *National Health Interview Survey,* Number of Persons Using Assistive Technology Devices, Table 1b, 2010. Retrieved from http://www.cdc.gov/nchs/nhis/ad292tb1.htm.

For those who use mobility devices on a daily basis, the majority are elderly, although a surprising number are working age. Many are unemployed and, as a result, are much more likely to live in poverty. Across the age range, persons with mobility impairments who use mobility devices tend to have lower wage earnings as well as lower educational success.

Interestingly enough, more women than men use mobility devices. African Americans are more likely to use mobility devices than whites, who are in turn much more likely than Asians and Pacific Islanders to be device users. Latinos are less likely to use mobility devices than people not of Hispanic origin.

Persons who use mobility devices, especially those using wheelchairs and scooters, are much more likely to see themselves as someone with a disability. This self-image may be due in large part to the tremendous number of access barriers they face every day. For example, homes with even a few stairs may keep some persons in wheelchairs locked within their own home. Accessible public transportation is often difficult to reach, and even when it is available, it may not work well for someone with a mobility impairment. Fatigue, timeliness of routes, and social embarrassment create numerous barriers for those with mobility impairments. Some people have difficulty moving about their home safely, or sometimes even from room to room, due to narrow doorways and halls. For many persons with mobility impairments, the difficulties can become overwhelming. Although environmental access has improved immensely since implementation of the Americans with Disabilities Act in 1990, substantial challenges remain.

AT for Communication

Accessible Media

Numerous advancements in media access have been made in the United States over the last 30 years. Accessible media includes access to images, text, video, and audio through a variety of outlets, including print and electronic materials. Accessible media aims to provide access for individuals with a variety of disabilities through alternate formats and accommodations. Within education, there is a growing need for timely and accurate delivery of accessible content. In 2007, the U.S. Department of Education provided funding for Bookshare to provide accessible textbooks free of charge to students with print disabilities.

AT for Vision and Hearing

Individuals with vision loss use AT to access their environment. Assistive technology for individuals with vision loss may include modifications to existing technologies, such as providing alternate formats or accommodations. Assistive technology is also available to meet the unique needs of individuals with low vision and blindness. For example, alternative formats for regular print materials can include Braille, large print, tape recordings, and electronic formats. Table 14 includes data on the use of AT by individuals with vision disabilities within the United States.

Hearing impairments are the most common form of chronic physical disability in the United States. Hearing loss may be mild or severe; it may be present at birth, occur throughout life, or appear during later years.

Table 14   Number of Persons Using Assistive Technology Devices Related to Vision, by Age of Person and Type of Device: United States, 1994

	All ages	44 years and under	45–64 years	65 years and over
Vision devices	Number in thousands			
Any vision device**	527	123	135	268
Telescopic lenses	158	40	49	70
Braille	59	*28	*23	*8
Readers	68	*15	*14	39
White cane	130	*35	48	47
Computer equipment	*34	*19	*8	*7
Other vision technology	277	51	76	151

Source: U.S. Centers for Disease Control, *National Health Interview Survey*, Number of Persons Using Assistive Technology Devices, Table 1d, 2010. Retrieved from http://www.cdc.gov/nchs/nhis/ad292tb1.htm

Notes: *Figure does not meet standard of reliability or precision. **Numbers do not add to these totals because categories are not mutually exclusive; a person could be counted more than once for any device type.

A hearing loss may present substantial educational, vocational, and social barriers or be a minor inconvenience. Individuals with hearing loss also benefit from numerous assistive technologies. Usage data is indicated in Table 15.

Prevalence of AT Use

In 1990, only 5% of the total population (or about a quarter of all people with disabilities) used any assistive devices.

Similarly, as Table 17 shows, relatively few American families report that their children with special health care needs are using assistive devices.

Overall assistive technology use in the United States today is difficult to estimate. Data from past surveys similar to the AT survey discussed here, such as the Disability Follow Back Survey (DFS) administered

Table 15   Number of Persons Using Assistive Technology Devices Related to Hearing, by Age of Person and Type of Device: United States, 1994

	All ages	44 years and under	45–64 years	65 years and over
Hearing devices	Number in thousands			
Any hearing device**	4,484	439	969	3,076
Hearing aid	4,156	370	849	2,938
Amplified telephone	675	73	175	427
TDD/TTY	104	58	*25	*21
Closed caption television	141	66	*32	43
Listening device	106	*26	*22	58
Signaling device	95	*37	*23	35
Interpreter	57	*27	*21	*9
Other hearing technology	93	*28	*24	41

Source: U.S. Centers for Disease Control, *National Health Interview Survey*, Number of Persons Using Assistive Technology Devices, Table 1c, 2010. Retrieved from http://www.cdc.gov/nchs/nhis/ad292tb1.htm.

Notes: *Figure does not meet standard of reliability or precision. **Numbers do not add to these totals because categories are not mutually exclusive; a person could be counted more than once for any device type.

Table 16   Usage of Assistive Devices in the United States, 1990

	Percentage	Estimated Number
Use AT	5.3%	13,128,000
Report unmet need for AT	1.0%	2,508,000
No reported AT use	93.7%	232,062,113
Total	100.0%	247,698,113

Source: LaPlante, M. P., Hendershot, G. E., & Moss, A. J., The prevalence of need for assistive technology devices and home accessibility features, *Technology and Disability, 6*, 17–28, 1997.

Table 17   Equipment Use by Children With Special Health Care Needs in the United States, 1995

Type of Equipment	Estimated Number
Breathing equipment	858,041
Mobility aid	204,787
Brace	166,806
Hearing aid	109,551
Self-care equipment (ADLs)	60,149
Hearing assistance equipment	38,459
Visual aid	24,066
Equipment for toileting or eating	18,613
Artificial limb	15,084

Source: Newacheck, P. W., Strickland, B., Shonkoff, J. P., Perrin, J. M., McPherson, M., McManus, M., et al., An epidemiologic profile of children with special health care needs, 1998, Pediatrics, 102(1), 117–23.

between 1994 and 1997, show that, based on a weighted sample of 41.8 million Americans with disabilities aged 18 years and older:

- 8.3 million Americans with disabilities needed special equipment or aids (AT) to perform basic activities of daily living (ADLs) such as bathing or showering, dressing, eating, getting in and out of bed or chairs, walking, getting outside, and using the toilet, including getting to the toilet.
- 15.4 million Americans with disabilities reported using assistive devices or technologies (primarily medical), such as tracheotomy tubes, ostomy bags, catheterization equipment, glucose monitors, diabetic equipment and supplies, inhalers, nebulizers, hearing aids, crutches, canes, walkers, wheelchairs, scooters, and feeding tubes.
- 16.6 million Americans with disabilities used special equipment, aids, or assistive technology (either one or more of the above).
- 7.4 million Americans with disabilities had surgical implants, such as shunts to drain away fluid, artificial joints, implanted lenses, pins, screws, nails, wires, rods, or plates, artificial heart valves, pacemakers, silicone implants, infusion pumps, implanted catheters, organ implants, and cochlear implants.

- 14 million Americans with disabilities lived in homes modified to meet their special needs. Among these, over 1.5 million persons reported needing further home modifications to already existing ones. An additional 1 million persons with disabilities who did not have any home modifications indicated that they needed such accommodations.
- 511,000 Americans with disabilities reported using modified cars or vans. Another 369,000 persons with disabilities reported needing modifications to their cars or vans. Of these, 60,000 persons needed modifications in addition to the ones they already had, and the remaining 309,000 persons used vehicles that had no modifications but needed them.
- 15.1 million Americans with disabilities worked at the time of the interview. In this group, 4.2 million persons reported being limited in the kind or amount of work they could do.
- 714,000 Americans with disabilities reported having an accessible work environment that included hand rails or ramps; accessible parking or an accessible transportation stop close to the building; elevators, including elevators designed for persons with special needs; specially adapted work stations; restrooms designed for persons with special needs; automatic doors; voice synthesizers; TDDs; infrared systems or other technical devices; Braille, enlarged print, special lighting, or audiotape devices; and special pens or pencils, chairs, or other office supplies.
- 1.3 million Americans with disabilities working at the time of the interview reported needing one or more of the above-mentioned workplace designs and accessories.
- 402,000 Americans with disabilities were provided with special accommodations that included readers, oral and sign language interpreters, job coaches, personal assistants, job redesign or slowing the pace of tasks, reduced work hours and more breaks, part-time work, and other types of equipment, help, and work arrangements not named above.
- 531,000 Americans with disabilities, working at the time of the interview, indicated a need for one or more of the previously mentioned special accommodations (Carlson, Ehrlich, Berland, & Bailey, 2001).

Due to the narrow scope of questions and the dated information provided by the survey data, these figures may substantially underestimate the full scope of AT use and need in the United States.

Public Access to AT

Although the benefits of AT are widely known, there are still numerous individuals with disabilities who do not receive the AT they need. A particular challenge occurs in isolated rural areas, where access to health care in general may be lacking. With the passage of the Americans with Disabilities Act in 1990 and Section 504 of the Rehabilitation Act in 1973, there have been increased requirements for physical and electronic accessibility in public places. Public libraries are one example of the type of institutions that are working to enhance the accessibility options for individuals. In 1997, however, only 4.3% of libraries nationwide provided public access to software or hardware for people with disabilities, as shown in Table 18.

Computer Usage

Computer use in the United States has expanded exponentially over the past decade. However, individuals with disabilities lag behind in their ownership and use of a computer and in their Internet access. In fact, less than one-quarter of people with a work disability have a computer at home, compared to more than half of people with no disability. Similarly, nondisabled people have Internet access from home at nearly three times the rate of people with a work disability, 31.1% to 11.4% (Kaye, 2000).

Equipment Recycling and Loan Programs

All 50 states, plus the District of Columbia and the five U.S. territories, reported having some kind of assistive technology device reutilization program in the 2008 and 2009 annual Assistive Technology Act reports to Congress. Table 19 presents more details about the types of programs offered.

Table 18   Percentage of Public Libraries With Public Access Software for People With Disabilities, by Type of Community

Type of Community	Percentage With Public Access Software
Urban	11.1%
Suburban	5.1%
Rural	3.0%
Overall	4.3%

Source: Bertot, J. C., McClure, C. R., & Fletcher, P. D., *The 1997 national survey of public libraries and the Internet: Summary results,* Washington, DC: American Library Association Office for Information Technology Policy, 1997.

Table 19   Types of AT Reutilization Programs

Type of Program	# of States 2008	# of States 2009
Exchange	43	36
Recycle/repair/refurbish	40	44
Open-ended loan	28	31

Source: U.S. Department of Education, Office of Special Education and Rehabilitative Services, Rehabilitation Services Administration, *Annual Report to Congress on the Assistive Technology Act of 1998 for Fiscal Years 2004 and 2005,* 2009. Retrieved from http://www2.ed .gov/about/reports/annual/rsa/atsg/2004/index.html

The reported cost savings to consumers in 2009 was $17,229,179, and 27,004 individuals were able to obtain technology through these programs. The 54 states and territories that reported having short-term device loan programs in place in 2009 made 37,833 AT loans to individuals. The majority of the loans (66%) were for the purpose of helping consumers to make decisions about what technology would benefit them. The remaining loans were for short-term accommodations, as shown in Table 20.

Table 20   Short-Term AT Device Loan Participants

Borrower	Percentage of Total Loans
Individuals with disabilities	38
Family members	17
Education representatives	22
Health, allied health, rehab reps	15

Source: U.S. Department of Education, Office of Special Education and Rehabilitative Services, Rehabilitation Services Administration, *Annual Report to Congress on the Assistive Technology Act of 1998 for Fiscal Years 2004 and 2005,* 2009. Retrieved from http://www2.ed.gov/about/reports/annual/rsa/atsg/2004/index.html.

A total of 51,415 assistive technology devices were loaned for an average of 35 days, as shown in Table 21.

Table 21   Types of AT Devices Borrowed Short-Term

Type of Device	Percentage
Learning and cognition	24
Speech and communication	20
Computers and related	11
Vision/hearing/mobility/daily living/ environmental/recreation	6–9

Source: U.S. Department of Education, Office of Special Education and Rehabilitative Services, Rehabilitation Services Administration, *Annual Report to Congress on the Assistive Technology Act of 1998 for Fiscal Years 2004 and 2005,* 2009. Retrieved from http://www2.ed .gov/about/reports/annual/rsa/atsg/2004/index.html.

Device Demonstrations

Under the Assistive Technology Act, states report how many assistive technology device demonstrations they do to help consumers, families, and service providers make decisions about the best technology to select for an individual. During the 2009 fiscal year, 55 states and territories reported conducting a total of 32,868 device demonstrations. Table 22 presents a breakdown of the types of AT devices included in these demonstrations.

Barriers to AT Nationally

Physical and communication barriers can limit access by people with disabilities to public buildings, sidewalks, and transportation systems. The evidence indicates, however, that many of these barriers have been removed since passage of the Americans with Disabilities Act. In 1993, for instance, 12,728 small businesses claimed a tax credit for "disabled access." This credit applies to removal of architectural barriers, hiring signers for hearing-impaired customers, and printing documents in Braille or large type or making them available on cassette.

Table 22   Types of AT Devices Demonstrated

Type of Device	Percentage
Hearing	18
Computers/related	17
Speech	14
Vision and daily living	13
Learning	10
Mobility	8
Recreation/environmental & vehicle	1–3

Source: U.S. Department of Education, Office of Special Education and Rehabilitative Services, Rehabilitation Services Administration, *Annual Report to Congress on the Assistive Technology Act of 1998 for Fiscal Years 2004 and 2005*, 2009. Retrieved from http://www2.ed.gov/about/reports/annual/rsa/atsg/2004/index.html.

Public transportation systems have become more accessible to riders with mobility or sensory impairments, as well. In 2005, the U.S. Department of Transportation estimated that 97% of public transit buses were wheelchair accessible—a 300% increase over the 24% that were accessible in 1985. In addition, 75% of people with disabilities interviewed in a 1994 Harris poll said that access to restaurants, theaters, stores, and museums had improved since the passage of the ADA.

Despite these clear signs of progress, a great many barriers continue to impede the full social participation of people with disabilities. One-quarter (24%) of the respondents to the 1994 Harris poll said that access to public buildings was a problem for them. Some modes of transportation, such as intercity buses and the New York subway system, remain almost totally inaccessible to those with limited mobility. Air travel can be partially accessible or completely inaccessible, depending on the type of plane and the presence or absence of a jetway. And only a tiny fraction (2.9% according to 1990 data from the NHIS) of Americans live in homes with any accessibility features, such as ramps, extra-wide doors, elevators, or stair lifts (Kaye, 1998).

Barriers to Social Participation

People with disabilities continue to live in relative social isolation. Among persons living in the community rather than in institutions, those with disabilities are twice as likely to live alone as those without disabilities (19.6% vs. 8.4%), according to data from the 1990 NHIS. Half (51%) of the respondents to the 1994 Harris poll of Americans with disabilities said that lack of a full social life was a problem for them (Kaye, 1998).

Figure 11   Rate of Participation in Social, Cultural, and Commercial Activities

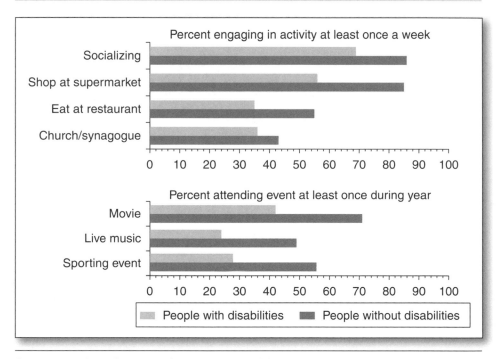

Source: Kaye, S., Is the status of people with disabilities improving?, Figure 3, UCSF Disability Statistics Center, 1998. Retrieved from http://dsc.ucsf.edu/figure.php?pub_id=7&section_id=1&figure_id=3.

AT Sales and Industry Data

The United States represents the largest market in the world for AT manufacturers and service providers. Domestic market demand accounted for 76.5% of the 1999 sales of U.S. companies that participated in an

AT survey completed by the National Institutes of Health (Brandt & Pope, 1997; Whyte, 1998). Older populations are growing rapidly in Western Europe and Asia, however, creating extensive opportunities for American AT companies to expand sales worldwide.

As reported elsewhere in this chapter, the aging population is growing rapidly throughout the world. As a result, the demand for assistive technologies and accessible mainstream technologies is also continuing to increase dramatically. U.S. Census data shows that 10% of the U.S. population that is between 18 and 34 years of age has some kind of disability, a percentage figure that continues to rise as Americans age. For Americans between 65 and 74 years of age, about 42% have a disability, while and 64% of people age 75 years or older cope with some sort of disability (U.S. Department of Commerce, 2000).

While many of the skills necessary to manufacture and sell AT devices are similar to those found in other industries, the AT market serves a smaller and often complex customer base. This factor creates difficulties for manufacturers seeking to hire individuals who can work with and understand the multiple demands placed on individuals with disabilities, their families, and service providers. For example, funding streams and billing requirements for the AT industry are complex at best. Employees need to have specialized knowledge of insurance reimbursement requirements and federal and state medical reimbursement programs. Similarly, AT product representatives must be knowledgeable about the variations in reimbursement levels of the 50 states and 6 territories to determine a product's actual cost to the end user. These specialized demands have created skills shortages in the AT industry, as Table 24 indicates.

Not only do AT manufacturers benefit from state and federal funding streams for equipment purchases by consumers, they also benefit from available research and development programs sponsored by the federal government. Small Business Innovation Research (SBIR) grants are available that (1) enable the production of intellectual property that companies can transform into products; and (2) provide a source of funds to enable manufacturers to take an idea from the conceptual stage through commercialization.

Research and development data is fractured at best, and information on how much federal funding is used in this way is difficult to obtain. However, a review of federal funding streams does show increases over time in the amount and availability of federal dollars for research and development of new ATs.

At the National Institutes of Health, for example, expenditures for AT research and development have climbed significantly over the years.

Table 23 Company Sales Revenues by World Market Region

	1997	1998	% Change 1997–1998	1999 (est.)	% Change 1998–1999
TOTAL	$2,354,358,592	$2,659,477,215	12.96%	$2,865,970,683	7.76%
United States	$1,856,378,902	$2,126,719,899	14.56%	$2,320,180,830	9.10%
Canada and Mexico	$68,728,724	$86,541,477	25.92%	$99,182,574	14.61%
Western Europe	$278,316,610	$285,911,535	2.73%	$282,131,864	-1.32%
Eastern Europe	$64,631,449	$57,232,404	-11.45%	$59,007,169	3.10%
South America	$12,925,206	$14,505,746	12.23%	$7,257,539	-49.97%
Central America	$923,344	$1,770,760	91.78%	$1,406,900	-20.55%
Middle East	$1,774,154	$2,362,504	33.16%	$2,181,313	-7.67%
Asia & Pac. Rim	$36,766,537	$37,898,850	3.08%	$43,981,226	16.05%
Africa	$1,499,946	$1,782,534	18.84%	$1,967,204	10.36%
Australia	$24,314,968	$25,548,868	5.07%	$25,120,800	-1.68%
Other	$8,098,753	$19,202,638	137.11%	$23,553,264	22.66%

Source: U.S. Department of Commerce, Bureau of Industry and Security, *Technology Assessment of the U.S. Assistive Technology Industry,* Table 1. Retrieved from http://www.bis.doc.gov/defenseindustrialbaseprograms/osies/defmarketresearchrpts/assisttechrept/5intro_ markets.htm#1.

Table 24   Reported AT Industry Skills Shortages*

Scientists, Engineers & Techs	Manufacturing & Assembly	Health Care Professionals
• Biomedical Engineers/ Designers • Computer Programmers • Digital Signal Processing (DSP) • New Product Design Engineers • Electrical Engineers • Electronics Designers and Techs • Fluid Engineers • Mechanical Engineers • Process Engineers • Software Developers/ Engineers	• Machinists • Computer Numerically Controlled (CNC) Machine Operators • Metal Fabricators • Mold Makers • Welders • Shoemakers • Sewing Machine Operators • Shop Floor Skills	• Certified Rehabilitation Techs • Occupational Therapists With Design/ Manufacturing Skills **Marketing/Sales/ General & Administrative** • Accountants • Billing/ Collection Skills • Product Representatives

Source: U.S. Department of Commerce, Bureau of Industry and Security, Technology Assessment of the U.S. Assistive Technology Industry, Table 18. Retrieved from http://www.bis.doc.gov/defenseindustrialbaseprograms/osies/defmarketresearchrpts/assisttechrept/20_attractingfolks.htm#18.

Note: *Based on comments from 89 of 357 survey participants.

Table 25   NIH Assistive Technology R&D Spending (Millions)

	FY 1998	*FY 1999*	*FY 2000*	*Change*
Total w/SBIR	$79.3	$100.4	$116.0	46%
Non SBIR	$59.8	$79.3	$94.8	58.5%
SBIR Only	$19.5	$21.1	$21.2	8%

Source: Strategy for the Development and Transfer of Assistive Technology and Universal Design, Interagency Committee on Disability Research, December 2000.

Total funding hit $116 million in fiscal year 2000, up from $100.4 million in 1999 and $79.3 million in 1998—a 46% increase for the two-year period. The National Science Foundation (NSF) allocated $8.6 million to a range of disability research projects, many of which are supportive of assistive technology; $900,000 of the NSF funds went to AT-specific R&D. The Department of Education, through the National Institute on Disability and Rehabilitation Research (NIDRR), allocated about $15.7 million to research and development in FY 2000; and the Department of Veterans Affairs research and development budget for assistive technology was $5.6 million (U.S. Department of Commerce, 2000).

Despite the benefits U.S. companies obtain from public spending for people with disabilities, the AT industry's relationship with federal and state agencies is less than optimal, according to survey participants. Numerous companies expressed frustration with the way federal and state government agencies conduct business. Some AT product manufacturers complained that often they must traverse a regulatory maze in order to take advantage of available funds.

Because government (Medicare/Medicaid) chooses specific technologies to fund through third-party payments for individual consumers, federal and state agencies are effectively the "market maker" for products. As a result, AT manufacturers reported they were often unable to create and market the technologies they felt would be most useful to their customers because they were not covered by insurance.

The AT industry is represented by hundreds of companies that sell almost 40,000 different products to a broad range of customers who can and do have very different needs. The American AT industry is comprised of large, medium, and small businesses producing a wide range of products intended for a frequently limited, sometimes regulated, and often partially subsidized market (U.S. Department of Commerce, 2000).

AT companies include those that develop, manufacture, distribute, and support products tailored—exclusively or in part—to the needs of persons with often very specific disabilities. Software, electronics, household items, medical supplies, furniture, enhancements to existing products, and specialized devices are just a few examples. To some extent, companies are aligned in industry subgroups, or categories of equipment, such as manufacturers that make devices for people with hearing disabilities, mobility devices such as wheelchairs, or AT products for people who are blind.

Sixty percent of the survey respondents reported fewer than 10 employees, a finding that suggests that in many instances AT industry workers may shoulder multiple responsibilities within their business unit. Survey data also indicate that it is not unusual for AT manufacturers and suppliers to produce a variety of products that serve multiple sectors of the AT market (U.S. Department of Commerce, 2000).

Most firms are primarily engaged in manufacturing, assembly, and distribution activities. Of the 287 firms that reported manufacturing as a primary or secondary activity, 245 of them stated that product distribution is also a primary or secondary function for their companies. Product assembly is a major, or secondary, role for 166 of the 359 survey participants. Some 141 firms disclosed that they count applied research and development activities as primary or secondary functions in their operations (U.S. Department of Commerce, 2000).

The AT product areas with the largest number of company participants (as shown in Figure 12) are: devices to aid mobility, 20.7%; orthotics/prosthetics, 12.2%; aids to daily living, 12%; and communications devices, 10.4%.

Figure 12   Product Areas of Surveyed American AT Companies

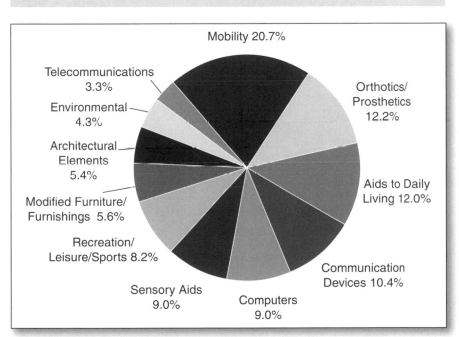

Source: U.S. Department of Commerce, Bureau of Industry and Security, *Technology Assessment of the U.S. Assistive Technology Industry,* Chart 1. Retrieved from http://www .bis.doc.gov/defenseindustrialbaseprograms/osies/defmarketresearchrpts/assisttechrept/ images/atchart1.jpg.

Conclusion

Data that fully describe the AT industry and the people served by industry, governments, and the private sector are fragmented, and locating that data is frustrating at best. There remains a clear and present need for solid and up-to-date information representing what is actually happening in the field of AT, including information on devices, services, funding, and evidence-based outcomes of the efficacy of AT devices and services. As noted here and elsewhere in this book, persons with disabilities are quickly increasing in number, in part because Americans are surviving traumatic illnesses and injuries more frequently; neonatal care has improved dramatically; and the mortality rates for illnesses and diseases that were once fatal have fallen substantially. At the same time as the demand for assistive technology and services is increasing, however, researchers and service providers are often unable to secure funding for critically important work. Federal and state funding streams for these efforts are constrained or decreasing due to the current economic status, yet AT devices and services have the potential to save the government, insurance companies, and individuals billions of dollars in health care costs.

New technologies and the rapid deployment of broadband, tablet technologies, robotics, and cell phones worldwide also contribute an interesting twist to the field of AT. It is clear that technology has the potential to facilitate improved independence for persons with disabilities. It is up to the field to demonstrate its impact.

References and Further Reading

Altman, J., Thurlow, M., & Vang, M. (2010). *2007 Annual report on participation, annual performance report: 2007–2008 state assessment data.* Minneapolis, MN: National Center on Educational Outcomes (NCEO).

Bausch, M. E., & Ault, M. J. (2005). *Nationwide use of assistive technology implementation plans.* Lexington, KY: National Assistive Technology Research Institute (NATRI), University of Kentucky.

Benedict, R. E., & Baumgardner, A. M. (2009). A population approach to understanding children's access to assistive technology. *Disability and Rehabilitation, 31*(7), 582–592.

Blair, M. E. (2007). *U.S. education policy and assistive technology: Administrative implementation.* Logan, UT: Center for Persons with Disabilities, Utah State University.

Brandt, E. N., & Pope, A. M. (1997). *Enabling America: Assessing the role of rehabilitation science and engineering.* Washington, DC: National Academies Press.

Carlson, D., Ehrlich, N., Berland, B. J., & Bailey, N. (2001). Assistive technology survey results: Continued benefits and needs reported by Americans with disabilities. National Center for the Dissemination of Disability Research. Retrieved from http://www.ncddr.org/products/researchexchange/v07n01/atpaper/

Christensen, L. L., Lazarus, S. S., Crone, M., & Thurlow, M. L. (2008). *2007 State policies on assessment participation and accommodations for students with disabilities (Synthesis report 69).* Minneapolis, MN: National Center on Educational Outcomes.

Derer, K., Polsgrove, L., & Rieth, H. (1996). A survey of assistive technology applications in schools and recommendations for practice. *Journal of Special Educational Technology, 13,* 62–80.

Early, D., & Winton, P. (2001). Preparing the workforce: Early childhood teacher preparation at 2- and 4-year institutions of higher education. *Early Childhood Research Quarterly, 16,* 285–306.

Erickson, W., Lee, C., & von Schrader, S. (2010). *Disability statistics from the 2008 American Community Survey (ACS).* Ithaca, NY: Cornell University Rehabilitation Research and Training Center on Disability Demographics and Statistics (StatsRRTC). Retrieved from http://www.disabilitystatistics.org

Judge, S., Floyd, K., & Wood-Fields, C. (2010). Creating a technology-rich learning environment for infants and toddlers with disabilities. *Infants & Young Children, 23*(2), 84–92.

Kaye, H. S. (2000). Computer and Internet use among people with disabilities. *Disability Statistics Report 13.* San Franscisco, CA: U.S. Department of Education, National Institute on Disability and Rehabilitation Research.

Kaye, S. (1998). Is the status of people with disabilities improving? San Francisco, CA: UCSF Disability Statistics Center. Retrieved from http://dsc.ucsf.edu/publication.php?pub_id=7

LaPlante, M. P., Hendershot, G. E., & Moss, A. J. (1997). The prevalence of need for assistive technology devices and home accessibility features. *Technology and Disability, 6,* 17–28.

Long, T., Woolverton, M., Perry, D. F., & Thomas, M. J. (2007). Training needs of pediatric occupational therapists in assistive technology. *American Journal of Occupational Therapy, 61*(3), 345–354.

Mann, W. C., Goodall, S., Justiss, M. D., & Tomita, M. (2002). Dissatisfaction and non-use of assistive devices among frail elders. *Assistive Technology, 14*(2), 130–39.

Mann, W., Hurren, D., Tomita, M., & Charvat, B. (1997). Comparison of the UB-RERC-Aging Consumer Assessments Study with the 1986 NHIS and the 1987 NMES. *Topics in Geriatric Rehabilitation, 13*(2), 32–41.

Moore, H. W., & Wilcox, M. J. (2006). Characteristics of early intervention practitioners and their confidence in the use of assistive technology. *Topics in Early Childhood Special Education, 26,* 15–23.

National Council on Disability. (1993). *Study on the financing of assistive technology devices and services for individuals with disabilities.* Retrieved from http://www .ncd.gov/publications/1993/Mar41993#tab4

Newacheck, P. W., Strickland, B., Shonkoff, J. P., Perrin, J. M., McPherson, M. McManus, M., et al. (1998). An epidemiologic profile of children with special health care needs. *Pediatrics, 102*(1), 117–23.

Russell, J. N., Hendershot, G. E., LeClere, F., Howie, L. J., & Adler, M. (1997). Trends and differential use of assistive technology devices: United States, 1994. *Advance Data from Vital and Health Statistics, 292.* Hyattsville, MD: National Center for Health Statistics.

Smith, F. A., Butterworth, J., Domin, D., & Hall, A. C. (2012). Data note: VR outcome trends and the recent decline in employment for VR customers with intellectual disabilities. *Data Note Series,* Institute for Community Inclusion, Paper 2. Retrieved from http://scholarworks.umb.edu/ici_datanote/2

U.S. Census Bureau. (2002). 2000 Census of Population and Housing, Summary File 3: Technical Documentation. Washington, DC: Author.

U.S. Department of Commerce, Bureau of Industry and Security. (2000). *Technology assessment of the U.S. assistive technology industry.* Retrieved from http://www .bis.doc.gov/defenseindustrialbaseprograms/osies/defmarketresearchrpts/ assisttechrept/24_govtindustfuture.htm#41st#41st

U.S. Department of Education, National Center for Education Statistics. (2012). *The condition of education: Mathematics performance (indicator 24–2012).* Retrieved from http://nces.ed.gov/programs/coe/indicator_mat.asp

U.S. Department of Education, Office of Special Education and Rehabilitative Services, Rehabilitation Services Administration. (2006). *Annual report to Congress on the Assistive Technology Act of 1998 for fiscal years 2004 and 2005.* Washington, DC: Author. Retrieved from http://www2.ed.gov/about/ reports/annual/rsa/atsg/2004/at-act-report-04–05.doc

U.S. Department of Education, Office of Special Education Programs. (2009). Twenty-eighth annual report to Congress on the implementation of the Individuals with Disabilities Education Act. Washington, DC: Author.

Von Schrader, S., Erickson, W. A., & Lee, C. G. (2010). *Disability statistics from the Current Population Survey (CPS).* Ithaca, NY: Cornell University Rehabilitation Research and Training Center on Disability Demographics and Statistics (StatsRRTC). Retrieved from http://www.disabilitystatistics.org

Wehmeyer, M. L. (1998). National survey of the use of assistive technology by adults with mental retardation. *Mental Retardation, 36*(1), 44–51.

Whyte, J. (1998). Enabling America: A report from the Institute of Medicine on rehabilitation science and engineering. *Archives of Physical Medicine and Rehabilitation, 79*(11), 1477–1480.

Wilcox, M. J., Dugan, L. M., Campbell, P. H., & Guimond, A. (2006). Recommended practices and parent perspectives regarding AT use in early intervention. *Journal of Special Education Technology, 21*(4), 7–16.

Six

Annotated List of Organizations and Associations

Cathy Bodine and Lorrie Harkness

This chapter provides an annotated list of organizations and associations that are involved in developing, supporting, or promoting the use of assistive technologies and services. The list is divided into the following categories: Government Agencies, Information and Advocacy Organizations, Research and Development Organizations, Professional Organizations, and Other Resources.

Government Agencies

National Center on Accessing the General Curriculum (NCAC)
40 Harvard Mills Square, Suite 3
Wakefield, MA 01880-3233
Telephone: (781) 245-2212; (781) 245-9320 TDD
Fax: (781) 245-5212
E-mail: cast@cast.org
Web site: http://www.cast.org/ncac
According to its Web site, the National Center on Accessing the General Curriculum (NCAC) is a collaborative endeavor to improve access, participation, and progress within

the general education curriculum. Some of the necessary elements for success include utilizing experts in universal design, advanced teaching practices, educational policy, and consensus building activities. NCAC is a project of the Center for Applied Special Technology (CAST), and it is funded by the U.S. Department of Education's Office of Special Education Programs (OSEP).

National Institutes of Health (NIH)

9000 Rockville Pike
Bethesda, MD 20892
Web site: http://www.nih.gov
The National Institutes of Health (NIH) is housed within the U.S. Department of Health and Human Services. NIH is composed of 27 institutes and centers, each focused on particular diseases or body systems. A number of the institutes and centers fund research relevant to disability and assistive technologies.

National Science Foundation (NSF)

4201 Wilson Boulevard
Arlington, VA 22230
Telephone: (703) 292-5111; (800) 877-8339 TDD; (703) 292-5090; (800) 281-8749
E-mail: info@nsf.gov
Web site: http://www.nsf.gov
The National Science Foundation (NSF) is an independent federal agency created by Congress in 1950 "to promote the progress of science; to advance the national health, prosperity, and welfare; to secure the national defense." With an annual budget of about $6.9 billion (FY 2010), it is the funding source for approximately 20% of all federally supported basic research conducted by America's colleges and universities, including research on augmentative and assistive technologies.

United States Access Board

1331 F Street, NW, Suite 1000
Washington, DC 20004-1111
Telephone: (202) 272-0080; (800) 872-2253; (202) 272-0082 TTY
Fax: (202) 272-0081; (800) 993-2822 TTY
E-mail: info@access-board.gov
Web site: http://www.access-board.gov
The Access Board is an independent federal agency devoted to accessibility for people with disabilities. Created in 1973 to ensure access to federally funded facilities, the board now operates as a leading source of information on accessible design. The Access Board has expanded its focus from the built environment to encompass transportation, telecommunication, and other electronic and information technology (ICT).

U.S. Department of Education (USDOE)

400 Maryland Avenue, SW, Mailstop PCP-6038
Washington, DC 20202
Telephone and fax: (202) 245-7323
Web site: http://www2.ed.gov

Originating in 1867 as a congressionally mandated office to collect data on school systems and teachers, the U.S. Department of Education (USDOE) became a Cabinet-level agency in 1980. Today it is responsible for establishing policy for educational administrators and for coordinating federal assistance to education, including special education services, across the nation. There are a number of offices and institutes within the USDOE designed to support its mission to "promote student achievement and preparation for global competitiveness by fostering educational excellence and ensuring equal access."

The Office of Special Education and Rehabilitative Services (OSERS) within the USDOE is particularly pertinent to assistive technology services. OSERS is host to the National Institute on Disability and Rehabilitation Research (NIDRR), the Office of Special Education Programs (OSEP), and the Rehabilitation Services Administration (RSA). Together these three entities work to improve the lives of persons with disabilities across the lifespan. The Institute of Education Sciences (IES), also housed within the USDOE, was established in 2002.

National Institute on Disability and Rehabilitation Research (NIDRR)

NIDRR works to improve life participation of individuals of all ages with disabilities. It does this through a combination of community-based research and programs designed to foster improved understanding and knowledge translation of the benefits of a variety of supports and services, including assistive technologies.

Office of Special Education Programs (OSEP)

OSEP is responsible for administering the Individuals with Disabilities Education Act (IDEA) and works to provide leadership and funding to states and local districts. OSEP also provides support to institutions of higher education working to provide preservice preparation of educators, special educators, and allied health and paraprofessionals working in early intervention and other educational facilities.

Rehabilitation Services Administration (RSA)

RSA administers a number of grant programs designed to support the employment and community independence aspirations of persons with disabilities. RSA also provides Title I formula grants to support individual state vocational rehabilitation (VR) programs across the nation and its territories. Assistive technology devices and services are supported throughout the RSA programs, including the State Grant for Assistive Technology Program (# 84.224A). This program supports state efforts to improve the provision of assistive technology to individuals with disabilities of all ages through comprehensive, statewide programs that are consumer responsive. The State Grant for Assistive Technology Program makes assistive technology devices and services more available and accessible to individuals with disabilities and their families. The program provides one grant to each of the states, the District of Columbia, Puerto Rico, and the outlying areas.

Information and Advocacy Organizations

Alexander Graham Bell Association for the Deaf and Hard of Hearing
3417 Volta Place, NW
Washington, DC 20007
Telephone: (202) 337-5220; (202) 337-5221 TTY
E-mail: info@agbell.org
Web site: http://www.agbell.org
The Alexander Graham Bell Association for the Deaf and Hard of Hearing helps families, health care providers, and education professionals understand childhood hearing loss and the importance of early diagnosis and intervention. Through advocacy, education, research, and financial aid, AG Bell helps to ensure that every child and adult with hearing loss has the opportunity to listen, talk, and thrive in mainstream society.

American Association on Intellectual and Developmental Disabilities (AAIDD)
(formerly known as the American Association on Mental Retardation [AAMR])
501 3rd Street, NW, Suite 200
Washington, DC 20001
Telephone: (202) 387-1968; (800) 424-3688
Web site: http://www.aaidd.org
With membership over 5,000 strong in the United States and in 55 countries worldwide, AAIDD is a leader in advocating quality of life and rights for those with intellectual disabilities. AAIDD promotes progressive policies, sound research, effective practices, and universal human rights for people with intellectual and developmental disabilities.

American Association of Retired Persons
601 E Street, NW
Washington, DC 20049
Telephone: (888) OUR-AARP (687-2277); (877) 434-7589 TTY;
(877) MAS-DE50 (627-3350) Spanish; +1 (202) 243-3525 International
E-mail: member@aarp.org
Web site: http://www.aarp.org
Founded in 1958, AARP is a nonprofit, nonpartisan membership organization that helps people aged 50 and over to improve the quality of their lives. AARP has offices in all

50 states, the District of Columbia, Puerto Rico, and the U.S. Virgin Islands. As a social welfare organization, as well as the nation's largest membership organization for people 50+, AARP is leading a revolution in the way people view and live life.

American Council of the Blind (ACB)

2200 Wilson Boulevard, Suite 650
Arlington, VA 22201
Telephone: (202) 467-5081; (800) 424-8666
Fax: (703) 465-5085
E-mail: info@acb.org
Web site: http://www.acb.org
The ACB strives to improve the well-being of all blind and visually impaired people by: serving as a representative national organization of blind people; elevating the social, economic, and cultural levels of blind people; improving educational and rehabilitation facilities and opportunities, cooperating with public and private institutions and organizations concerned with blind services; encouraging and assisting all blind persons to develop their abilities; and conducting a public education program to promote greater understanding of blindness and the capabilities of blind people.

American Foundation for the Blind (AFB)

2 Penn Plaza, Suite 1102
New York, NY 10121
Telephone: (212) 502-7600
Fax: (888) 545-8331
E-mail: afbinfo@afb.net
Web site: http://www.afb.org
AFB is a national nonprofit that expands possibilities for the more than 25 million people with vision loss in the United States. AFB's priorities include broadening access to technology; elevating the quality of information and tools for the professionals who serve people with vision loss; and promoting independent and healthy living for people with vision loss by providing them and their families with relevant and timely resources. AFB's work in these areas is supported by its strong presence in Washington, D.C., ensuring that the rights and interests of Americans with vision loss are represented in public policies.

American Society on Aging (ASA)

71 Stevenson Street, Suite 1450
San Francisco, CA 94105-2938
Telephone: (415) 974-9600; (800) 537-9728
Fax: (415) 974-0300
E-mail: info@asaging.org
Web site: http://www.asaging.org

Founded in 1954, the American Society on Aging is an association of diverse individuals bound by a common goal: to support the commitment and enhance the knowledge and skills of those who seek to improve the quality of life of older adults and their families. The membership of ASA is a multidisciplinary array of professionals who are concerned with the physical, emotional, social, economic, and spiritual aspects of aging. They include practitioners, educators, administrators, policymakers, business people, researchers, students, and more.

American Society for Deaf Children (ASDC)
800 Florida Avenue, NE, #2047
Washington, DC 20002
Telephone: (800) 942-2732; (866) 895-4206
Fax: (410) 795-0965
E-mail: asdc@deafchildren.org
Web site: http://www.deafchildren.org
Founded in 1967 as a parent-helping-parent network, ASDC is a national, independent, nonprofit network with core values that believe a deaf or hard-of-hearing child is entitled to full communication access at home, at school, and in the community.

Arc of the United States
1660 L Street, NW, Suite 301
Washington, DC 20036
Telephone: (202) 534-3700; (800) 433-5255
Fax: (202) 534-3731
E-mail: info@thearc.org
Web site: http://www.thearc.org
The Arc of the United States is the largest community-based organization of and for people with intellectual and developmental disabilities. It provides an array of services and support for families and individuals and includes over 140,000 members affiliated through more than 730 state and local chapters across the nation. The Arc is devoted to promoting and improving supports and services for all people with intellectual and developmental disabilities.

Arthritis Foundation
P.O. Box 7669
Atlanta, GA 30357-0669
Telephone: (404) 872-7100; (800) 283-7800
Web site: http://www.arthritis.org
The Arthritis Foundation is the largest private, not-for-profit contributor to arthritis research in the world, funding more than $380 million in research grants since its founding

in 1948. It is the only national organization that supports the more than 100 types of arthritis and related conditions. Headquartered in Atlanta, the Arthritis Foundation has multiple service points located throughout the country. The foundation helps people take control of arthritis by providing public health education; pursuing public policy and legislation; and conducting evidence-based programs to improve the quality of life for those living with arthritis.

Autism Society of America

4340 East-West Highway, Suite 350

Bethesda, MD 20814

Telephone: (800) 328-8476

Web site: http://www.autism-society.org

The Autism Society of America is the nation's leading grassroots autism organization. It improves the lives of all people affected by autism by increasing public awareness about the day-to-day issues faced by people on the spectrum, advocating for appropriate services for individuals across the lifespan, and providing the latest information regarding treatment, education, research, and advocacy.

Better Hearing Institute (BHI)

1444 I Street, NW, Suite 700

Washington, DC 20005

Telephone: (800) 327-9355 V/TTY; (202) 216-9646

E-mail: mail@betterhearing.org

Web site: http://www.betterhearing.org

BHI is a not-for-profit corporation that educates the public about the neglected problem of hearing loss and what can be done about it. Founded in 1973, it is working to: erase the stigma and end the embarrassment that prevents millions of people from seeking help for hearing loss; show the negative consequences of untreated hearing loss for millions of Americans; promote treatment; and demonstrate that this is a national problem that can be solved.

Brain Injury Association of America (BIAA)

1608 Spring Hill Road, Suite 110

Vienna, VA 22182

Telephone: (703) 761-0750

Fax: (703) 761-0755

Web site: http://www.biausa.org

Founded in 1980, the Brain Injury Association of America is the leading national organization serving and representing individuals, families, and professionals who are touched by a life-altering, often devastating, traumatic brain injury (TBI). Together with its network of more than 40 chartered state affiliates, as well as hundreds of local chapters and support groups across the country, the BIAA provides information, education, and support to assist the 3.17 million Americans currently living with traumatic brain injury and their families.

Council for Exceptional Children (CEC)

1110 North Glebe Road, Suite 300
Arlington, VA 22201
Telephone: (888) 232-7733; (703) 620-3660; (866) 915-5000 TTY
Fax: (703) 264-9494
E-mail: service@cec.sped.org
Web site: http://www.cec.sped.org
The Council for Exceptional Children (CEC) is the largest international professional organization dedicated to improving the educational success of individuals with disabilities and/or gifts and talents. CEC advocates for appropriate governmental policies, sets professional standards, provides professional development, advocates for individuals with exceptionalities, and helps professionals obtain conditions and resources necessary for effective professional practice.

Council for Exceptional Children, Technology and Media (TAM) Division

2900 Crystal Drive, Suite 1000
Arlington, VA 22202-3557
E-mail: contactus@tamcec.org
Web site: http://www.tamcec.org
TAM is the official membership division of the Council for Exceptional Children that works to promote the availability and effective use of technology and media for individuals with exceptional learning needs. TAM member benefits include online access to the Journal of Special Education Technology (JSET) *and the* TAM Connector *(pdf) newsletter. TAM also hosts or co-sponsors occasional professional development events on assistive technology.*

Easter Seals

233 South Wacker Drive, Suite 2400
Chicago, IL 60606
Telephone: (312) 726-6200; (800) 221-6827; (312) 726-4258 TTY
Fax: (312) 726-1494
Web site: http://www.easterseals.com
Easter Seals has been helping individuals with disabilities and special needs, and their families, live better lives for nearly 90 years. From child development centers to physical

rehabilitation and job training for people with disabilities, Easter Seals offers a variety of services to help people with disabilities address life's challenges and achieve personal goals.

Family Voices, Inc.
2340 Alamo, SE, Suite 102
Albuquerque, NM 87106
Telephone: (505) 872-4774; (888) 835-5669
Fax: (505) 872-4780
Web site: http://www.familyvoices.org
Family Voices aims to achieve family-centered care for all children and youth with special health care needs and/or disabilities. Through a national network, the organization provides families with tools to make informed decisions, advocates for improved public and private policies, builds partnerships among professionals and families, and serves as a trusted resource on health care.

International Dyslexia Association (IDA)
40 York Road, 4th Floor
Baltimore, MD 21204
Telephone: (410) 296-0232
Fax: (410) 321-5069
Web site: http://www.interdys.org
IDA is a 501(c) (3) nonprofit, scientific, and educational organization dedicated to the study and treatment of the learning disability dyslexia, as well as related language-based learning differences. It is the oldest such organization in the United States serving individuals with dyslexia, their families, and professionals in the field with more than 10,000 members.

International Society for Technology in Education (ISTE)
1710 Rhode Island Avenue, NW, Suite 900
Washington, DC 20036
Telephone: (866) 654-4777 (U.S. & Canada); (202) 861-7777 (International)
Fax: (202) 861-0888
E-mail: iste@iste.org
Web site: http://www.iste.org/welcome.aspx
ISTE is the premier membership association for educators and education leaders engaged in improving teaching and learning by advancing the effective use of technology in grades PK-12 and teacher education. Home of the National Educational Technology Standards (NETS) and ISTE's annual conference and exposition (formerly the National Education Computing Conference [NECC]), ISTE represents more than 100,000 professionals worldwide.

International Society for Technology in Education (ISTE), Special Education Technology Special Interest Group (SETSIG)
1710 Rhode Island Avenue, NW, Suite 900
Washington, DC 20036
Telephone: (866) 654-4777 (U.S. & Canada); (202) 861-7777 (International)
Fax: (202) 861-0888
E-mail: iste@iste.org
Web site: http://www.iste.org/connect/special-interest-groups/sig-direc
tory/setsig.aspx
SETSIG seeks to provide leadership, policy development, resources, and training for members and serve as a catalyst for engaging the special education community within ISTE. Members work individually as well as collaboratively to conduct activities including workshops, trainings, webinars, and other professional development events. SETSIG has a number of different ways to get involved, from engaging in topical discussions to resource sharing via online social networking sites like Twitter and Delicious.

Learning Disabilities Association of America (LDA)
4156 Library Road
Pittsburgh, PA 15234-1349
Telephone: (412) 341-1515
Fax: (412) 344-0224
Web site: http://www.ldanatl.org
As the largest nonprofit volunteer organization advocating for individuals with learning disabilities, LDA has over 200 state and local affiliates in 42 states and Puerto Rico. LDA's international membership of over 15,000 includes members from 27 countries around the world.

Composed of individuals with learning disabilities, family members, and concerned professionals, the membership advocates for the almost three million students of school age with learning disabilities and for adults affected with learning disabilities.

National Association of the Deaf (NAD)
8630 Fenton Street, Suite 820
Silver Springs, MD 20910
Telephone: (301) 587-1788; (301) 587-1789 TTY
Fax: (301) 587-1791
Web site: http://www.nad.org
The National Association of the Deaf (NAD) is the nation's premier civil rights organization of, by, and for deaf and hard-of-hearing individuals in the United States. Established in 1880, the NAD was shaped by deaf leaders who believed in the right of the American deaf community to use sign language, to congregate on issues important to its members, and to have its interests represented at the national level. These beliefs remain in place to this day, with American Sign Language as a core value.

National Autism Association (NAA)

1330 West Schatz Lane

Nixa, MO 65714

Telephone: (877) 622-2884

E-mail: naa@nationalautism.org

Web site: http://www.nationalautismassociation.org

The NAA educates and empowers families affected by autism and other neurological disorders, while advocating on behalf of those who cannot fight for their own rights. It identifies funding efforts for research on finding a cure for the neurological damage from which so many affected by autism suffer.

National Center for Learning Disabilities (NCLD)

381 Park Avenue South, Suite 1401

New York, NY 10016

Telephone: (212) 545-7510; (888) 575-7373

Fax: (212) 545-9665

Web site: http://www.ncld.org

The NCLD provides essential information to parents, professionals, and individuals with learning disabilities, promotes research and programs to foster effective learning, and advocates for policies to protect and strengthen educational rights and opportunities. Since its beginning, NCLD has been led by passionate and devoted parents committed to creating better outcomes for children, adolescents, and adults with learning disabilities.

National Dissemination Center for Children with Disabilities (NICHCY)

1825 Connecticut Avenue, NW, Suite 700

Washington, DC 20009

Telephone: (202) 884-8200; (800) 695-0285

E-mail: nichcy@aed.org

Web site: http://www.nichcy.org

NICHCY serves the nation as a central source of information on: disabilities in infants, toddlers, children, and youth; IDEA, which is the law authorizing special education; No Child Left Behind (as it relates to children with disabilities); and research-based information on effective educational practices.

Paralyzed Veterans of America

801 18th Street, NW

Washington, DC 20006

Telephone: (202) 416-7710; (800) 555-9140

E-mail: info@pva.org

Web site: http://www.pvaorg.com

Paralyzed Veterans of America works to maximize the quality of life for its members and all people with spinal cord injury/disease (SCI/D) as a leading advocate for health care, SCI/D research and education, veterans' benefits and rights, accessibility and the removal of architectural barriers, sports programs, and disability rights.

Post-Polio Health International (PHI)
4207 Lindell Boulevard, #110
St. Louis, MO 63108-2915
Telephone: (314) 534-0475
Fax: (314) 534-5070
Web site: http://www.post-polio.org
Polio survivors, like individuals from other disability communities, require lifelong intermittent intervention. Many chronically ill individuals have the dual challenge of managing their complex conditions while also negotiating innumerable obstacles to accessing quality health care. Post-Polio Health International's mission is to enhance the lives and independence of polio survivors and home ventilator users through education, advocacy, research, and networking.

Special Education Technology Special Interest Group (SETSIG)
See International Society for Technology in Education (ISTE), Special Education Technology Special Interest Group (SETSIG)

Technology and Media (TAM)
See Council for Exceptional Children, Technology and Media (TAM) Division

United Cerebral Palsy (UCP)
1660 L Street, NW, Suite 700
Washington, DC 20036
Telephone: (800) 872-5827
Fax: (202) 776-0414
E-mail: info@ucp.org
Web site: http://www.ucp.org
For 60 years, United Cerebral Palsy (UCP) has been committed to change and progress for persons with disabilities. Founded in 1949, the national organization and its nationwide network of affiliates strive to ensure the inclusion of persons with disabilities in every facet of society—from the Web to the workplace, from the classroom to the community. As one of the largest health charities in America, the mission of United Cerebral Palsy is to advance the independence, productivity, and full citizenship of people with disabilities.

United States Society for Augmentative and Alternative Communication (USSAAC)
100 E. Pennsylvania Avenue, Courtyard
Towson, MD 21286
E-mail: info@ussaac.org
Web site: http://www.ussaac.org
The United States Society for Augmentative and Alternative Communication is the national chapter of ISAAC, the International Society for Augmentative and Alternative Communication. The organization is dedicated to supporting the needs and desires of people who use AAC, as well as the larger community of professionals, manufacturers, and family members.

Research and Development Organizations

ASSIST
Center for Assistive Technology and Environmental Access (CATEA)
Georgia Institute of Technology
490 Tenth Street
Atlanta, GA 30332-0156
Telephone: (404) 894-4960 V/TTY
Fax: (404) 894-9320
E-mail: catea@coa.gatech.edu
Web site: http://www.assistivetech.net
ASSIST is a searchable online database for assistive technology with a mission to provide access to information on AT devices and services as well as other community resources for people with disabilities and the general public. The site is created and maintained through the collaboration of the Georgia Tech Center for Assistive Technology and Environmental Access (CATEA), the National Institute on Disability and Rehabilitation Research (NIDRR), and the Rehabilitation Services Administration (RSA).

Assistive Technology Partners
601 E. 18th Avenue, Suite 130
Denver, CO 80203
Telephone: (303) 315-1280; (800) 225-3477; (303) 837-8964 TTY
Fax: (303) 837-1208
E-mail: ATP@ucdenver.edu
Web site: http://www.Assistivetechnologypartners.org
Assistive Technology Partners is a program within the Department of Physical Medicine and Rehabilitation, School of Medicine, University of Colorado-Anschutz Medical Campus,

and encompasses programs in four major areas: Clinical Services, Outreach and Information Services, Research and Engineering, and Education. Their mission is for persons with cognitive, sensory, and/or physical disabilities to reach their highest potential at home, school, work, and play through the addition of appropriate assistive technologies to their lives.

Assistive Technology Research Institute (ATRI)
Misericordia University
301 Lake Street
Dallas, PA 18612
Telephone: (570) 674-6413
E-mail: atri@misericordia.edu
Web site: http://atri.misericordia.edu
Located at Misericordia University, ATRI is a regional resource to provide information and education in the application of assistive technology and universal design principles to allow individuals with limited function to participate in their personal lives and their communities to the greatest extent possible. The Institute's activities include research into the usability of devices and products that are specifically marketed to allow individuals with disabilities improved function (assistive technologies) and products that are intended for the general population, but have been designed to be usable by people with functional restrictions as well as able-bodied individuals.

Center for Applied Special Technology (CAST)
40 Harvard Mills Square, Suite 3
Wakefield, MA 01880-3233
Telephone: (781) 245-2212; (781) 245-9320 TTY
Fax: (781) 245-5212
E-mail: cast@cast.org
Web site: http://www.cast.org
CAST is a nonprofit research and development organization that works to expand learning opportunities for all individuals, especially those with disabilities, through Universal Design for Learning.

Center on Disabilities, California State University Northridge (CSUN)
18111 Nordhoff Street
Bayramian Hall 110
Northridge, CA 91330
Telephone: (818) 677-2578
Fax: (818) 677-4929
Web site: http://www.csun.edu/cod
The Center on Disabilities assists Cal State Northridge students in realizing their academic and career goals. A team of disability and educational specialists are available to

students on a year-round basis. In addition, students may receive training on assistive technology, access the help of peer mentors, and participate in the wide range of cultural and social activities offered at the university. The annual internationally recognized assistive technology conference provides training programs to expand the knowledge base of professionals and introduce newcomers to the disability field.

Center for Universal Design
College of Design
North Carolina State University
Campus Box 8613
Raleigh, NC 27695-8613
Telephone: (919) 515-3082; (800) 647-6777
Fax: (919) 515-8951
Email: cud@ncsu.edu
Web site: http://www.design.ncsu.edu/cud
The Center for Universal Design is a national research, information, and technical assistance center that evaluates, develops, and promotes accessible and universal design in housing, buildings, outdoor and urban environments, and related products. The Center's work manifests the belief that all new environments and products, to the greatest extent possible, should be usable by everyone regardless of their age, ability, or circumstance. Part of the College of Design at North Carolina State University (NCSU) in Raleigh, the Center promotes the concept of universal design in all design, construction, and manufacturing disciplines through research, design assistance, and training.

Coleman Institute for Cognitive Disabilities
University of Colorado System
3825 Iris Avenue, Suite 200
Boulder, CO 80301
Telephone: (303) 492-0639
Fax: (303) 735-5643
Web site: http://www.colemaninstitute.org
The Coleman Institute for Cognitive Disabilities was established in 2001 by the Regents of the University of Colorado. The Institute's mission is to catalyze and integrate advances in science, engineering, and technology to promote the quality of life and independent living of people with cognitive disabilities.

Media Access Group at WGBH
One Guest Street
Boston, MA 02135
Telephone: (617) 300-3600 V/TTY
Fax: (617) 300-1020

E-mail: access@wgbh.org

Web site: http://main.wgbh.org

The Media Access Group at WGBH pioneered and delivered captioned and described media for over 30 years to people in their homes, classrooms, at work, and in the community. The Media Access Group continues to develop new solutions to access challenges as technology, and the way people consume media, evolves.

National Assistive Technology Research Institute (NATRI)

Department of Special Education and Rehabilitation Counseling

229 Taylor Education Building

University of Kentucky

Lexington, KY 40506-0001

Telephone: (859) 257-4713; (859) 257-4714 TDD

Fax: (859) 257-1325

Web site: http://natri.uky.edu

NATRI conducts research related to the planning, development, implementation, and evaluation of assistive technology (AT) services in schools, identifies promising practices in the delivery of AT services, and disseminates research findings and information that will assist school personnel to develop or improve AT policies and practices for students with disabilities.

National Center for Technology Innovation (NCTI)

1000 Thomas Jefferson Street, NW

Washington DC 20007

Telephone: (202) 403-5323; (202) 333-3072 TTY

Fax: (202) 403-5001

E-mail: ncti@air.org

Web site: http://www.nationaltechcenter.org

NCTI advances learning opportunities for individuals with disabilities by fostering technology innovation. Specifically, NCTI helps researchers, product developers, manufacturers, and publishers to create and commercialize products of value to students with special needs.

To achieve its goals NCTI offers services to: analyze needs, issues, trends, and promising technology innovations; cultivate a collaborative network; promote reliable research-based solutions; and facilitate successful commercialization approaches for the education market.

Quality Indicators for Assistive Technology Services (QIAT)

University of Kentucky Computing Center

128 McVey Hall

Lexington, KY 40506

Telephone: (859) 257-2900

Fax: (859) 323-1978

E-mail: listmaster@lsv.uky.edu

Web site: http://natri.uky.edu/assoc_projects/qiat/index.html

The QIAT Consortium is a nationwide grassroots group that includes hundreds of individuals who provide input into the ongoing process of identifying, disseminating, and implementing a set of widely applicable Quality Indicators for Assistive Technology Services in School Settings that can be used as a tool to support school districts, assistive technology service providers, consumers of assistive technology services, universities, professional developers, and policy makers as they attempt to develop judicious and equitable policies related to assistive technology services.

Professional Organizations

American Occupational Therapy Association (AOTA)

4720 Montgomery Lane

P.O. Box 31220

Bethesda, MD 20824-1220

Telephone: (301) 652-2682; (800) 377-8555 TDD

Fax: (301) 652-7711

Web site: http://www1.aota.org

AOTA was established in 1917 to represent the interests and concerns of occupational therapy practitioners and students of occupational therapy and to improve the quality of occupational therapy services.

American Physical Therapy Association (APTA)

1111 North Fairfax Street

Alexandria, VA 22314-1488

Telephone: (800) 999-APTA (2782); (703) 684-APTA (2782); (703) 683-6748 TDD

Fax: (703) 684-7343

Web site: http://www.apta.org

APTA is a national professional organization representing more than 74,000 members. Its goal is to foster advancements in physical therapy practice, research, and education.

American Speech-Language-Hearing Association (ASHA)

2200 Research Boulevard

Rockville, MD 20850

Telephone: (301) 296-5700; (800) 638-8255; (301) 296-5650 TTY

Fax: (301) 296-5650
E-mail: actioncenter@asha.org
Web site: http://www.asha.org
ASHA is the professional, scientific, and credentialing association for 140,000 members and affiliates who are speech-language pathologists, audiologists, and speech, language, and hearing scientists in the United States and internationally. Its goal is to make effective communication—a human right—accessible and achievable for all.

Assistive Technology Industry Association (ATIA)
401 North Michigan Avenue
Chicago, IL 60611-4267
Telephone: (312) 321-5172; (877) OUR-ATIA (687-2842)
Fax: (312) 673-6659
E-mail: info@ATIA.org
Web site: http://www.atia.org
A not-for-profit membership organization of manufacturers, sellers, and providers of technology-based assistive devices and/or services, ATIA represents the interests of its members to business, government, education, and the many agencies that serve people with disabilities. Its mission is to serve as the collective voice of the assistive technology industry so that the best products and services are delivered to people with disabilities.

Association of Assistive Technology Act Programs (ATAP)
700 McKnight Park Drive, Suite 708
Pittsburgh, PA 15237
Telephone: (202) 643-ATAP (2827)
E-mail: atap@ataporg.org
Web site: http://www.ataporg.org
ATAP was established in 1997 to provide support to statewide Assistive Technology (AT) program members to enhance the effectiveness of AT programs on the state and local level, and to promote the national network of AT programs. ATAP facilitates the coordination of state AT programs nationally and provides technical assistance and support to its members. ATAP represents the needs and interests of the state AT programs and is the national voice of the AT programs.

Association for Special Education Technology (ASET)
P.O. Box 10018
RPO Watline
Mississauga ON L4Z 4G5
Canada
Web site: http://www.aset-ontario.ca

ASET is a new and growing network of adaptive and assistive technology consultants, teachers, technicians, and support staff from educational institutions across Ontario who are dedicated to the support of students with special needs through the use of technology.

International Society for Augmentative and Alternative Communication (ISAAC)
49 The Donway West, Suite 308
Toronto ON M3C 3M9
Canada
Telephone: +1 (416) 385-0351
Fax: +1 (416) 385-0352
Web site: http://www.isaac-online.org
Working to improve the life of every child and adult with speech difficulties, ISAAC started in 1983 and has thousands of members in 50 countries. Members are people who use augmentative and alternative communication, their families, therapists, teachers, doctors, researchers, and people who make communication aids.

Rehabilitation Engineering and Assistive Technology Society of North America (RESNA)
1700 North Moore Street, Suite 1540
Arlington, VA 22209-1903
Telephone: (703) 524-6686
Fax: (703) 524-6630
E-mail: membership@resna.org
Web site: http://resna.org
RESNA's purpose is to improve the potential of people with disabilities to achieve their goals through the use of technology. The society serves that purpose by promoting research, development, education, advocacy, and provision of technology; and by supporting the people engaged in these activities. RESNA's membership ranges from rehabilitation professionals to consumers to students. All members are dedicated to promoting the exchange of ideas and information for the advancement of assistive technology.

Other Resources

Alliance for Technology Access (ATA)
1119 Old Humboldt Road
Jackson, TN 38305
Telephone: (731) 554-5282; (731) 554-5283 TTY; (800) 914-3017
Fax: (731) 554-5283
Web site: http://www.ataccess.org

ATA supports access to and innovation in technology tools for people with disabilities by developing a network of AT Centers providing assessment, education, and support for people with disabilities, their families, and disability-related professionals. The ATA Online Community (AOC) is a place for everyone to participate in trainings, forums, and opportunities to dialog with experts. The ATA Services Directory connects people to tools and services in communities worldwide. Funding comes from foundation and corporate grants, contracts, membership fees, donations, fees for services, and publications.

Closing The Gap
526 Main Street
P.O. Box 68
Henderson, MN 56044
Telephone: (507) 248-3294
Fax: (507) 248-3810
Web site: http://www.closingthegap.com
Closing The Gap, Inc. is an organization that focuses on assistive technology for people with special needs through its bimonthly magazine, annual international conference, and extensive Web site.

Family Center on Technology and Disability (FCTD)
Academy for Educational Development (AED)
1825 Connecticut Avenue, NW, 7th Floor
Washington, DC 20009-5721
Telephone: (202) 884-8068
Fax: (202) 884-8441
E-mail: fctd@aed.org
Web site: http://www.fctd.info
FCTD is a resource designed to support organizations and programs that work with families of children and youth with disabilities. FCTD offers a range of information and services on the subject of assistive and instructional technologies.

Family Village
Waisman Center
University of Wisconsin-Madison
1500 Highland Avenue
Madison, WI 53705-2280
E-mail: familyvillage@waisman.wisc.edu
Web site: http://www.familyvillage.wisc.edu
A Web site for children and adults with disabilities, their families, and their friends and allies, Family Village brings together thousands of online resources in an organized,

easy-to-use directory. The centerpiece of Family Village is the library, where visitors can find information on over 300 diagnoses. Visitors can also learn about assistive technology, legal rights and legislation, special education, leisure activities, and much more.

Journal of Special Education Technology (JSET)

Department of Educational Psychology, Special Education Program
University of Oklahoma
820 Van Vleet Oval, Room 326
Norman, OK 73019
Telephone: (405) 325-1533
Fax: (405) 325-7661
E-mail: jset@ou.edu
Web site: http://www.tamcec.org/jset

JSET is a refereed professional journal that presents up-to-date information and opinions about issues, research, policy, and practice related to the use of technology in the field of special education. JSET supports the publication of research and development activities, provides technological information and resources, and presents important information and discussion concerning important issues in the field of special education technology to scholars, teacher educators, and practitioners.

National Center on Deafness (NCOD)

California State University-Northridge
18111 Nordhoff Street
Chisholm Hall, Mail Drop 8267
Northridge, CA 91330-8267
Telephone: (818) 677-2611 V/TTY
Fax: (818) 677-7192
E-mail: ncod@csun.edu
Web site: www.csun.edu/ncod

The Center on Deafness was established in 1972 as an administrative coordinating unit for the deaf programs on the California State University-Northridge campus. By 1978 the achievements of the center's alumni and students had begun to have national impact and the name of the Center on Deafness was changed to the National Center on Deafness. Approximately 200 deaf and hard-of-hearing students attend CSUN each semester and register through the National Center on Deafness to receive services such as interpreting, real-time captioning, typewell, note taking, tutoring, and academic advisement.

National Rehabilitation Information Center (NARIC)

8201 Corporate Drive, Suite 600
Landover, MD 20785

Telephone: (800) 346-2742; (301) 459-5984 TTY
E-mail: naricinfo@heitechservices.com
Web site: http://www.naric.com
As a leader in providing interactive information to the disability and rehabilitation community, NARIC's Web site continues this tradition by putting the information into the hands of the users through online publications, searchable databases, and timely reference and referral data.

Special Education and Technology Connections (SET Connections)
P.O. Box 3872
Barrington, IL 60010
Telephone: (847) 732-3823
E-mail: info@SETConnections.org
Web site: http://www.setconnections.org
The purpose of SET Connections is educational: to promote an overall understanding of technology and its benefits and to assist in utilizing technology to improve the field of education, with an emphasis on special education. The organization initiates and encourages ideas and activities which support this endeavor. Membership is open to all who are interested in promoting and learning about the use of technology in education.

Seven

Selected Print and Electronic Resources

Cathy Bodine and Maureen Melonis

This chapter provides resources for further learning in the field of assistive technology. It is organized in two sections, print and electronic resources, and further separated into categories by disability. Each resource listed includes a brief description indicating why this resource is included. Both print and electronic resources were selected for their value to students and lay readers as they explore the field of assistive technology on their research journey. Older publications were included when the information they provided was particularly relevant to the learner or when they were highly cited publications. Categories include

Print Resources	Electronic Resources
General Information on Assistive Technology	General Information on Assistive Technology
AT for Infants, Toddlers, and Young Children	AT and the Law/Legislation
AT and Education	AT Research
AT and Employment	Funding

(Continued)

(Continued)

Print Resources	Electronic Resources
AT Assessment and Abandonment	Universal Design
AT Outcomes	Inclusion
AT and Communication	Academic Application Ideas 　　Math 　　Reading 　　Writing 　　Science 　　Social Studies
AT and Motor Issues	Autism
AT and Vision Loss	Vision
AT and Hearing	Hearing
AT and Cognitive Disability	Communication
	Early Childhood
	Access Issues/Motor
	Computers
	Switch Use
	Organizational/Time-Saving Strategies

Print Resources

General Information on Assistive Technology

Braddock, D., Hemp, R., & Rizzolo, M. C. (2008). *The state of the states in developmental disabilities: 2008.* Washington, DC: American Association on Intellectual and Developmental Disabilities.
　　Updated annually, this comprehensive publication provides an overview of programmatic trends for individuals with developmental disabilities living in the United States. This volume provides a detailed reference on public spending and revenue for programs and services for individuals with developmental disabilities.

Cook, A. M., & Miller-Polgar, J. (2007). *Cook and Hussey's assistive technologies: Principles and practice* (3rd ed.). St. Louis, MO: Mosby-Year Book.

This leading textbook in AT is utilized in graduate courses throughout the world. It provides a wealth of information on AT and is well supported with illustrations. It is a must read for those aspiring to attain the Assistive Technology Practitioner Certification in the United States.

Olson, D. A., & Deruyter, F. (Eds.). (2001). *Clinician's guide to assistive technology* (1st ed.). St. Louis, MO: Mosby.
For the healthcare professional interested in AT, this valuable resource is divided into five sections, which provide a comprehensive overview for all ages and disabilities. Over 40 contributing authors from the field provided input to this text.

Paciello, M. G. (2000). *Web accessibility for people with disabilities.* Lawrence, KS: CMP Books.
Designed for Web site designers and IT administrators seeking information on evaluating Web site accessibility and building accessible user interfaces, this exhaustive resource provides information on Web accessibility.

Pape, T. L.-B., Kim, J., & Weiner, B. (2002). The shaping of individual meanings assigned to assistive technology: A review of personal factors. *Disability and Rehabilitation, 24*(1–3), 5.
This literature review explores the influence of individual meanings on AT use. Results indicate that cultural factors and psychosocial influences shape individual meanings. It offers a resource to substantiate the integration of AT through the exploration of meanings assigned to devices, expectations, and anticipated social costs.

Robitaille, S. (2010). *The illustrated guide to assistive technology and devices: Tools and gadgets for living independently.* New York, NY: Demos Health.
With timely information on AT options for independent living, this resource explores a wide range of technologies. It focuses on the use of AT to increase independence while offering real-world examples of AT applications.

Sullivan, J., Kelker, K. A., & Holt, R. (2000). *Family guide to assistive technology.* Brookline, MA: Brookline Books.
This practical, easy-to-read book is designed as a tool for parents and caregivers seeking additional resources on AT for children. It contains a synopsis of technologies, manufacturers, and vendors, as well as strategies for acquisition.

AT for Infants, Toddlers, and Young Children

Campbell, P., Milbourne, S., Dugan, L., & Wilcox, M. (2006). A review of evidence on practices for teaching young children to use assistive technology devices. *Topics in Early Childhood Special Education, 26*(1), 3–13.

This literature review is cited frequently, as it summarizes 104 articles that address AT for young children published between 1980 and 2004. It addresses the scarcity of relevant published literature in the field.

Dugan, L., Campbell, P., & Wilcox, M. (2006). Making decisions about assistive technology with infants and toddlers. *Topics in Early Childhood Special Education, 26*(1), 25–32.
A comprehensive overview of the assessment process when selecting AT for young children, this article is a valuable resource for clinicians and families. Barriers to AT selection and use are provided.

Hutinger, P. L., Bell, C., & Daytner, G. (2006). Establishing and maintaining an early childhood emergent literacy technology curriculum. *Journal of Special Education Technology, 21*(4), 39–54.
This three-year study examined the impact of literacy curriculum incorporating AT implementation in preschool classrooms. The study found a positive impact of technology use to increase access to literacy. Benefits were found for children with disabilities, correlated with increased length of time teachers used the curriculum.

Judge, S. (2006). Constructing an assistive technology toolkit for young children: Views from the field. *Journal of Special Education Technology, 21*(4), 17–24.
In a summary of the field of early intervention and AT, the authors discuss the implementation of an AT toolkit to address these barriers. This article is often referred to by early intervention providers serving young children.

Lane, S. J., & Mistrett, S. (2002). Let's play! Assistive technology interventions for play. *Young Exceptional Children, 5*(2), 19–27.
This publication summarizes an intervention model for incorporating AT into play. The importance of AT in play and matching the families' values and lifestyle is emphasized. The study found that when this method was implemented, play became more complex and interactive.

Long, T., Huang, L., Woodbridge, M., Woolverton, M., & Minkel, J. (2003). Integrating assistive technology into an outcome-driven model of service delivery. *Infants & Young Children, 16*(4), 272–283.
This study highlights the importance of AT intervention for young children and provides a review of relevant literature exploring barriers to intervention. An outcomes-driven model was applied within a 10-step framework to guide service providers in assessing AT needs. It is a valuable resource for clinicians providing early intervention AT services.

Moore, H., & Wilcox, M. (2006). Characteristics of early intervention practitioners and their confidence in the use of assistive technology. *Topics in Early Childhood Special Education, 26*(1), 15–23.

Summarizing results of an AT survey of confidence given to early intervention providers, this article explores the correlation between a provider's level of confidence in their skill set and understanding of AT with AT selection, acquisition, and implementation.

Wilcox, M., Dugan, L. M., & Campbell, P. H. (2006). Recommended practices and parent perspectives regarding AT use in early intervention. *Journal of Special Education Technology, 21*(4), 7–16.
This study found that many parents of young children with disabilities evaluated and acquired AT without provider assistance, and that they perceived the devices as having limited success. The study emphasized the importance of provider and family collaboration in the selection and implementation of AT. It is recommended reading for those learning to deliver AT assessments in early intervention.

AT and Education

Beard, L. A., Bowden-Carpenter, L., & Johnston, L. (2010). *Assistive technology: Access for all students* (2nd ed.). Englewood Cliffs, NJ: Prentice Hall.
This second edition provides an informative discussion of universal design for learning for individuals working with students with disabilities in the classroom.

Bowser, G., & Reed P. (1995). Education TECH points for assistive technology planning. *Journal of Special Education Technology, 12*(4), 325–338.
Describing a method for school district teams to utilize when delivering AT services, this article continues to influence assistive technology service delivery throughout the United States, despite the date of publication. It addresses AT implementation process from initial referral to implementation and review.

Bugaj, C. R., & Norton-Darr, S. (2010). *The practical (and fun) guide to assistive technology in public schools: Building or improving your district's AT team.* Eugene, OR: International Society for Technology in Education.
This recent publication by the International Society for Technology in Education addresses the integration of assistive technology in the classroom setting. Authors include step-by-step guidelines for organizing and implementing a school AT team.

Dell, A., Newton, D., & Petroff, J. (2007). *Assistive technology in the classroom: Enhancing the school experiences of students with disabilities.* Upper Saddle River, NJ: Pearson Education.
Containing practical applications of AT in the classroom, this book emphasizes the natural inclusion of AT in the academic curriculum as well as in communication with teachers. A variety of technology options are addressed for individuals with a range of disabilities.

Edyburn, D., Higgins, K., & Boone, R. (Eds.). (2005). *The handbook of special educa-tion technology research and practice*. Whitefish Bay, WI: Knowledge by Design.
This informative reference book contains research and practice recommendations for technology in education. The book features 41 chapters organized in 8 sections with over 100 authors. It is recommended reading for teachers, related service personnel, and administrators in special education.

Sze, S., & Cowden, P. (2009). *Assistive technology in special education and rehabilita-tion*. San Diego, CA: University Readers.
This book assists education professionals in including AT into the daily curriculum for students with a variety of disabilities. It provides numerous examples to ensure the needs of the student are adequately addressed.

Zabala, J., Bowser, G., Blunt, M., Hartsell, K., Carl, D., Korsten, J., & Reed, P. (2000). Quality indicators for assistive technology services in school settings. *Journal of Special Education Technology, 15*(4), 25–36.
This influential work continues to guide the implementation of AT in the schools. The QIAT (Quality Indicators for Assistive Technology Services) consortium designed this tool to assist professionals and families in eight areas of consideration in the assessment and implementation of AT services.

AT and Employment

De Jonge, D., Scherer, M., & Rodger, S. (2007). *Assistive technology in the workplace*. St Louis, MO: Mosby Elsevier.
This book provides an overview of the process for selecting, integrating, and utilizing AT in the work environment. Stages of the process are explained and methods to address barriers are presented. Case studies of AT applications in the workplace are incorporated with results of an assistive technology user study.

Fuhrer, M. J. (2003). A framework for the conceptual modeling of assistive technol-ogy device outcomes. *Disability and Rehabilitation, 25*(22), 1243.
This highly cited article seeks to develop a conceptual framework for the planning of AT outcome research. A literature review of unmet needs of the framework is offered, followed by assumptions and framework implications. The authors identify factors which impact AT outcomes, including the device type, its user, and their environment.

Langton, A. J. (2001). Enhancing employment outcomes through job accommoda-tion and assistive technology resources and services. *Journal of Vocational Rehabilitation, 16*(1), 27.
The authors explore the importance of AT applications for individuals with disabili-ties in employment settings. A case is made for the inclusion of AT into the work setting to enhance employment outcomes.

Lazzaro, J. J. (2001). *Adaptive technologies for learning & work environments.* (2nd ed.). Chicago, IL: ALA Editions.

This comprehensive resource on AT and employment provides complex information in a non-technical format. The book features information on assistive technology devices and services and includes a detailed list of resources. The second edition contains 10 chapters that address the assistive technology needs of individuals with a wide variety of disabilities, including learning, sensory, physical, and communication disabilities.

Phillips, B., & Zhao, H. (1993). Predictors of assistive technology abandonment. *Assistive Technology, 5,* 36–45.

This study analyzed why individuals with disabilities accept or reject AT. A survey of 227 adults indicated abandonment rates at 29.3%, with mobility aids ranked highest. The study found four factors most often related to abandonment. These included: lack of user consideration in device selection, easy device procurement, poor performance of device, and change in user needs.

Wehmeyer, M. L., Palmer, S. B., Smith, S. J., Parent, W., Davies, D. K., & Stock, S. (2007). Technology use by people with intellectual and developmental disabilities to support employment activities: A single-subject design meta-analysis. *Journal of Vocational Rehabilitation, 24*(2), 81–86.

The authors conducted a meta-analysis which found potential benefits of AT for employment and rehabilitation of individuals with intellectual and developmental disabilities. The study emphasized the importance of universal design and a need for more research in this area.

AT Assessment and Abandonment

Alliance for Technology Access. (2004). *Computer resources for people with disabilities: A guide to exploring today's assistive technology* (4th ed.). Alameda, CA: Hunter House.

This fourth-edition book continues to be a favorite among individuals with disabilities, their family members, and those who work with them. It is divided into three sections. The first section provides an overview of the AT selection process, including setting goals and identifying user preferences. The second section offers information to help the user explore considerations in selecting a device. Finally, the third section provides AT resources, including legislative information, funding sources, vendors, and organizations.

Galvin, J., & Scherer, M. J. (1996). *Evaluating, selecting and using appropriate assistive technology.* Gaithersburg, MD: Aspen.

Although dated, this often-cited, seminal work highlights best practices in the evaluation, selection, and acquisition of AT for individuals with disabilities. In addition to

AT applications for home, school, work, and recreation, legal issues and funding are addressed. Authors include leading field experts, many of whom have disabilities themselves, adding a personal perspective on the assessment process.

Scherer, Marcia J. (1996). Outcomes of assistive technology use on quality of life. *Disability and Rehabilitation, 18*(9), 439.
Despite the date of publication, this article continues to offer guiding principles for the field of AT, emphasizing consumer involvement in the decision-making process. It addresses the high rate of abandonment of AT devices by end users and summarizes research. The literature supports the matching of person and technology while considering environment, user preference, and device features.

AT Outcomes

King, T. (1999). *Assistive technology—Essential human factors.* Boston: Allyn & Bacon.
This innovative book proposed a new framework for consideration in AT assessment. King emphasized four factors associated with technology use or abandonment, including motivation to do the task, physical effort, cognitive effort, and time involved. He was the first to indicate the correlation between these factors and the ability to predict device success.

Scherer, M. J. (2001). *Assistive technology: Matching device and consumer for successful rehabilitation.* Washington, DC: American Psychological Association.
This informative book provides guidelines for rehabilitation professionals to collaborate with individuals with disabilities around assistive technology evaluation and implementation. Evidence-based practices are emphasized, as is the process for matching the needs of the consumer to the appropriate device.

Scherer, M. J. (2005). *Living in the state of stuck: How assistive technology impacts the lives of people with disabilities* (4th ed.). Cambridge, MA: Brookline Books.
The fourth edition of this book provides a rich exploration of the impact of AT on individuals with disabilities from 1985 to 2004. Scherer includes sections on relationship rehabilitation and reports on the Matching Persons with Technology Tool.

AT and Communication

Beukelman, D. R., & Mirenda, P. (2006). *Augmentative and alternative communication: Supporting children and adults with complex communication needs* (3rd ed.). Baltimore, MD: Paul Brookes.
This seminal textbook, now in its third edition, is a must read for individuals seeking critical information on augmentative and alternative communication (AAC) assessment and intervention. It includes an overview of the field and addresses AAC for all ages

and disabilities. It provides a wealth of theoretical knowledge cited in the literature as well as evidence-based service delivery models and implementation guides.

Millar, D., Light, J., & Schlosser, R. (2006). The impact of augmentative and alternative communication intervention on the speech production of individuals with developmental disabilities: A research review. *Journal of Speech Language Hearing Research, 49,* 248–264.
Providing a meta-analysis of literature between 1975 and 2003 to identify the impact of augmentative and alternative communication (AAC) on speech production, this article summarizes early research in the field. Results indicated no evidence for a decrease in speech production following the implementation of AAC. To the contrary, gains in speech production were noted. It is cited frequently as a resource for families (and practitioners) who may be apprehensive about beginning an AAC intervention because of concerns that it will prevent the child from developing traditional speech.

Schlosser, R. W. (2003). *The efficacy of augmentative and alternative communication: Toward evidence-based practice.* San Diego, CA: Academic Press.
Schlosser discusses evidence-based practice (EBP) for the field of augmentative and alternative communication (AAC). The book provides a history of EBP, followed by a summary of current research in the field. Levels of evidence in terms of hierarchy are discussed and needs in the field identified. It is recommended for those new to the field seeking an overview of relevant AAC literature.

AT and Motor Issues

Batavia, M. (2009). *The wheelchair evaluation: A clinician's guide* (2nd ed.). Boston, MA: Jones & Bartlett.
This second edition adds relevant industry updates to a valuable reference on the assessment process for wheelchair selection for individuals with disabilities. Written by a physical therapist, this book provides a valuable tool for practicing clinicians as well as students new to the clinical decision-making process of evaluations. It covers an overview of the evaluation process, including selection of wheelchair components, fitting, ethical issues, funding, and documentation. It is essential reading for those completing wheelchair evaluations.

Mann, W. C., Ottenbacher, K. J., Fraas, L., Tomita, M., & Granger, C. V. (1999). Effectiveness of assistive technology and environmental interventions in maintaining independence and reducing home care costs for the frail elderly: A randomized controlled trial. *Archives of Family Medicine, 8,* 210–217.
This randomized control study indicates the importance of assistive technology to slow the decline of function in the elderly. It examined the impact of environmental interventions and assistive technology on the independence of 104 home-based frail

elderly individuals. The authors conclude that the rate of decline of functional independence for frail elderly can be slowed through the application of AT and environmental interventions.

Russell, J. N., Hendershot, G. E., LeClere, F., & Howie, L. J. (1997). Trends and differential use of assistive technology devices: United States, 1994. *Advance Data from Vital & Health Statistics, 292.* Hyattsville, MD: National Center for Health Statistics.
Although dated, this report from the U.S. Department of Health, Education, and Welfare presents data on the use of assistive technology devices in the United States for vision, mobility, hearing, and orthopedic impairments. The study found positive correlations in use of AT, particularly for the aging. It is frequently cited by professionals in the field.

AT and Vision Loss

Abner, G. H., & Lahm, E. A. (2002). Implementation of assistive technology with students who are visually impaired: Teachers' readiness. *Journal of Visual Impairment & Blindness, 96*(2), 98–105.
Students with vision impairment benefit from AT in the educational environment. This article summarizes the opinions of teachers of students with visual impairments and addresses student AT use and barriers. It provides a case for the ongoing professional development needs of teachers.

Hersh, M. A., & Johnson, M. A. (Eds.). (2008). *Assistive technology for visually impaired and blind people.* New York, NY: Springer-Verlag.
Designed for students, healthcare workers, and engineers, this informative book explains the physiology of the visual system while exploring potential devices to address the needs of the visually impaired. It presents practical applications for development and implementation as well as engineering and design principles used in AT development for the visually impaired and blind.

Kulyukin, V., Gharpure, C., Nicholson, J., & Osborne, G. (2006). Robot-assisted wayfinding for the visually impaired in structured indoor environments. *Autonomous Robots, 21*(1), 29–41.
This article addresses the use of robotics to assist individuals with vision impairments in wayfinding tasks. It provides a summary of implementation in indoor environments along with successes and challenges and recommendations for future research.

Presley, I. (2009). *Assistive technology for students who are blind or visually impaired: A guide to assessment.* New York, NY: AFB Press.
This book, written and published by the American Federation for the Blind, addresses the assistive technology needs of students who are visually impaired and blind.

It provides information on the entire process from AT assessment to implementation for students, as well as a comprehensive overview of current technology devices and services for both print and electronic information.

AT and Hearing

Carney, A. E. (1998). Treatment efficacy: Hearing loss in children. *Journal of Speech, Language, and Hearing Research, 41*(1), S61.
This article analyzes the treatment of children with hearing loss. It provides a clear definition of hearing loss, including the impact of hearing loss. A discussion of pertinent research is provided.

Dalton, D. S. (2003). The impact of hearing loss on quality of life in older adults. *The Gerontologist, 43*(5), 661.
The authors studied the impact of hearing loss on quality of life in older adults. Results indicated that the severity of hearing loss correlated with hearing handicap as well as self-reported communication difficulties.

Hersh, M. A., Johnson, M. A., Anderson, C., & Campbell, D. (2003). *Assistive technology for the hearing-impaired, deaf, and deaf/blind*. New York, NY: Springer.
This book addresses the complex technology needs of those with significant sensory impairment. It addresses legal and policy issues, as well as technology solutions for this population. A thorough background of the ear and eye is provided to help the reader understand the physiology of the disability. Chapters include a question-and-answer format with real-world applications and resources.

AT and Cognitive Disability

Bodine, C. (2005). Cognitive impairments, information technology systems, and the workplace. *Accessibility and Computing, 83*, 25–29.
The author provides an overview of cognitive disabilities in terms of diagnosis, prevalence, and causes and conditions. She also provides a summary of potential AT and a perspective for future research.

Bodine, C., & Scherer, M. J. (2006). Evaluation of cognitively accessible software to increase independent access to cell phone technology for people with intellectual disability. Technology for improving cognitive function. A workshop sponsored by the U.S. Interagency Committee on Disability Research (ICDR): Reports from working groups. *Disability and Rehabilitation, 28*(24), 1567–71.
This report summarizes the work of the U.S. Federal Interagency Committee on Disability Research (ICDR) on their task to provide strategic direction for the future of technology for persons with cognitive disabilities.

LoPresti, E. F., Bodine, C., & Lewis, C. (2007). Assistive technology for cognition. *IEEE Engineering and Medicine and Biology Magazine, 27*(2), 29–39.
This article highlights the challenges of cognitive disabilities and the potential applications of assistive technology to address those challenges.

Stock, S. E., Davies, D. K., Wehmeyer, M. L., & Palmer, S. B. (2008). Evaluation of cognitively accessible software to increase independent access to cell phone technology for people with intellectual disability. *Journal of Intellectual Disability Research, 52*(12), 1155.
Authors in this article explore the accessibility needs of individuals with cognitive disabilities within cell phone technology. In this study a multimedia interface for cell phone access prototype was designed and evaluated. Promising evidence of universal design for development of cell phone technology is discussed.

Wehmeyer, M. L. (1999). Assistive technology and students with mental retardation: Utilization and barriers. *Journal of Special Education Technology, 14*(1), 48–58.
This article summarizes the results of a comprehensive survey of over 500 family members of individuals with mental retardation to determine AT trends. Results were significant in that there was a significant population of individuals who could benefit from AT but did not have access.

Wehmeyer, M. L., Palmer, S., Smith, S. J., Davies, D., & Stock, S. (2007). The efficacy of technology use by people with intellectual disability: A single-subject design meta-analysis. *Journal of Special Education Technology, 23*(3).
This comprehensive literature review explores the benefits of technology for employment and rehabilitation for individuals with intellectual disabilities and the impact of technology use on employment-related outcomes. Results revealed an effective use of technology to promote outcomes for this population.

Electronic Resources

General Information on Assistive Technology

AbleData. Retrieved from http://www.abledata.com
AbleData is a database of information on assistive technology and rehabilitation equipment available in the United States. It contains a searchable database of more than 36,000 products. The site is maintained for the National Institute on Disability and Rehabilitation Research (NIDRR).

Assistive Technology Training Online (ATTO). Retrieved from http://atto.buffalo.edu

ATTO provides information on AT applications for students with disabilities. This site offers a free, simple online training for assistive technology. It also features tutorials on software. It is sponsored by the Center for Assistive Technology, University of Buffalo.

Disability.Gov. Retrieved from http://www.disability.gov
Disability.gov is an excellent federal resource on all things related to disability. Individuals can subscribe to this site for research and legislative updates.

Family Center on Technology and Disability. Retrieved from http://www.fctd.info
This interactive site contains a number of resources for families, providers, and others interested in instructional and assistive technology.

LearningPort. Retrieved from http://www.learningport.us
This valuable resource provides a professional development library of learning modules, webinars, and video resources funded by the U.S. Department of Education, Office of Special Education Programs (OSEP), to support the use of American Recovery and Reinvestment Act (ARRA) funds in states and local educational agencies (LEAs). These modules were developed to enable school teams to meet their increasing professional development needs. Search for assistive technology to find more than 20 online training resources.

QIAT. Retrieved from http://www.qiat.org
The Quality Indicators for Assistive Technology Services (QIAT) Web site offers a number of resources on quality indicators for AT service delivery in the schools. It includes a listserv with information and discussion regarding AT.

Trace Research and Development Center. Retrieved from http://trace.wisc.edu
This site contains a library of disability documents and resources and suggested guidelines for designing a wide variety of technologies. There are online searchable databases of AT products as well as freeware and shareware to download.

AT and the Law/Legislation

IDEA 1997. Retrieved from http://www.ed.gov/offices/OSERS/IDEA/the_law.html
This Web site provides an overview of the Individuals with Disabilities Education Act and is an excellent resource for learning about the laws around assistive technology and education.

IDEA 2004. McFassel, L. (2006). IDEA 2004's impact on AT applications in schools. *DATI AT Messenger, 14*(4). Retrieved from http://www.dati.org/newsletter/issues/2006n4/idea.html

This electronic article provides a summary of the changes in the 2004 re-authorization of the Individuals with Disabilities Education Act with regard to assistive technology.

National Assistive Technology Advocacy Project. Retrieved from http://www .nls.org/natmain.htm
This federally funded project is operated by Neighborhood Legal Services, Inc. The site contains information on funding AT, legislative decisions relating to AT, legal rulings, articles, etc. Their quarterly newsletter, the AT Advocate, offers valuable and timely updates for families and providers.

AT Research

Center for Implementing Technology in Education (CITEd). Retrieved from http://www.cited.org
CITEd is a technical assistance center designed to integrate instructional technology for all students to achieve high educational standards. The free registration allows access to free online training and literature updates by e-mail. It offers a vehicle to bookmark and tag resources, build and distribute custom toolkits, and comment on resources and other materials.

Journal of Special Education Technology (JSET). Retrieved from http://www.tamcec .org/jset
This professional, refereed journal provides research focused on the application of technology in the field of special education.

National Rehabilitation Information Center (NARIC). Retrieved from http:// www.naric.com
This comprehensive Web site offers a wealth of disability information, including resources on AT. The site contains over 70,000 documents and journal articles. The largest database, REHABDATA, contains numerous resources from the National Institute on Disability and Rehabilitation (NIDRR) to rehabilitation research and services.

Research Institute on Assistive Technology and Education. Retrieved from http:// natri.uky.edu
This site offers a portal with current research findings on the use of AT in education. The online AT planner is particularly valuable.

What Works Clearinghouse (WWC). Retrieved from http://ies.ed.gov/ncee/wwc
The clearinghouse collects, screens, and identifies studies of effectiveness of educational interventions (programs, products, practices, and policies). It aims to provide education consumers with high-quality reviews of the effectiveness of replicable educational interventions.

Funding

Neighborhood Legal Services, Inc. Hager, R. M., & Smith, D. (2003). *The public school's special education system as an assistive technology funding source: The cutting edge*. National Assistive Technology Advocacy Project. Retrieved from http://www.nls.org/specedat.htm
This booklet offers resources for funding of AT.

Universal Design

National Center on Accessing the General Curriculum. Retrieved from http://www.cast.org/ncac
This Web site enables users to learn about universal design and research-based tools.

National Center to Improve Practice in Special Education through Technology, Media, and Materials. Retrieved from http://www2.edc.org/NCIP/library/toc.htm
The NCIP maintains a library with resources about technology and special education.

Universal Design Education Online. Retrieved from http://www.udeducation.org
This Web site is a resource for those interested in teaching about universal design and accessibility. This new project, funded by the National Institute on Disability and Rehabilitation Research, is compiling educational materials related to universal design for download and use by others.

Inclusion

Going to College. Retrieved from http://www.going-to-college.org
This Web site contains information about attending college with a disability. It is designed for high school students and provides video clips, activities, and resources that can help in planning for college. It includes video interviews with college students with disabilities and activity modules to help students learn about themselves, what to expect from college, and to equip them with important considerations and tasks to complete when planning for college.

TAM (Technology and Media Division, Council for Exceptional Children). Retrieved from http://tam.uky.edu
This site offers access to the resources for integrating instruction about technology into special education developed by TAM's Technology Instructional Resource Initiative.

Academic Application Ideas

Georgia Project for Assistive Technology. Retrieved from http://atto.buffalo.edu/registered/DecisionMaking/resourceroom-docs/GPATparticipation.pdf

This document provides information on modifications, accommodations, and assistive technology solutions that may be implemented to support participation of students with disabilities in typical classroom activities.

National Center to Improve Practice in Special Education. Retrieved from http://www2.edc.org/NCIP/library/ec/Profile5.htm
This Web site contains examples of how AT can aid children with their development in the classroom. Included are descriptions of many different types of hardware to boost children's autonomy by allowing them to develop decision-making skills, participate in class discussions, gain literacy skills, and learn consequences to their actions.

Parents Let's Unite for Kids. Retrieved from http://www.pluk.org/AT1.html
This site was developed by parents in collaboration with the Federation for Children. It is designed to help parents learn about AT and the benefits to children with disabilities. It contains a list of considerations when using AT, evaluation steps, hints for parents, case studies, etc. Also included are resources on funding for assistive technologies, such as how to apply for funding, and tips that lead to success.

Math

National Library of Virtual Manipulatives. Retrieved from http://nlvm.usu.edu/en/nav/vlibrary.html
The National Library of Virtual Manipulatives (NLVM) was created through funding from an NSF grant that began in 1999 to develop a library of uniquely interactive, Web-based, virtual manipulatives or concept tutorials, mostly in the form of Java applets, for mathematics instruction (K–12 emphasis). There are numerous resources (bar graphs, abacus, fractions, etc.) that can be easily customized for math instruction.

Texas School for the Blind and Visually Impaired. Retrieved from http://www.tsbvi.edu/math
This Web site offers links to numerous adaptive tools and other math products for students with vision loss.

Reading

Bookshare. Retrieved from http://www.bookshare.org
Through federal funding from the U.S. Department of Education, this resource provides accessible books and periodicals. Bookshare offers free access for U.S. students with qualifying print disabilities. Members receive access to over 70,000 digital books, textbooks, periodicals, and other resources.

International Children's Digital Library Foundation. Retrieved from http://www
.childrenslibrary.org/index.shtml
*The mission of the foundation is to increase the ability of children to understand the
value of tolerance and respect for diverse cultures, languages, and ideas by making
the best in children's literature available online. Although there is not an option for
audio, books are available in many languages.*

LD Resources. Retrieved from http://www.ldresources.com
*This site has evolved over the years and now contains lists of tools, schools, organiza-
tions, professionals, and other resources for individuals with learning disabilities, as
well as new articles and commentaries. It also serves as a tremendous blog on learning disabilities. It hosts a collection of resources on various aspects of learning disabilities with comments from community members.*

Project Gutenberg. Retrieved from http://www.gutenberg.org
*Project Gutenberg is the first and largest single collection of free electronic books,
or E-books. It offers a library of 17,000 free E-books whose copyright has expired in
the United States. Books are downloadable to a computer so they can be read by a
screen reader.*

Reading Rockets. Retrieved from http://www.readingrockets.org
*Reading Rockets is a national multimedia project offering information and resources
on how young kids learn to read, why so many struggle, and how caring adults can
help. The Web site includes numerous strategies, resources, and research articles.*

Storyline Online. Retrieved from http://www.storylineonline.net
*The Screen Actors Guild Foundation features famous actors reading stories aloud
online. Stories have captioning options as well as numerous follow-up activities to
develop literacy.*

Tar Heel Reader. Retrieved from http://tarheelreader.org
*With a collection of free, easy-to-read, accessible books that can be speech-enabled and
accessed using multiple interfaces, this site offers rich resources for individuals with
disabilities. The books may be downloaded as slideshows in PowerPoint, Impress, or
Flash format.*

Writing

Education Place Graphic Organizers. Retrieved from http://www.eduplace.com/
graphicorganizer
*This link contains numerous graphic organizer ideas. The site gives users permission
to print and share them.*

Ghotit Contextual Speller. Retrieved from http://www.ghotit.com

This Web site is designed to provide free, online spelling assistance specifically for individuals with dyslexia. It boasts a 90% correction success. It is available for Windows with Internet Explorer only.

Jan Brett's Web Site. Retrieved from http://www.janbrett.com

Jan Brett is a famous children's illustrator. Her Web site contains numerous activities to promote literacy. There are many onscreen computer games with talking activities.

Science

Edheads. Retrieved from http://www.edheads.org

This site is run by a nonprofit organization that provides free, high-quality educational activities on the Web at no cost to students or teachers. Check out the virtual knee surgery, the simple machines, and the crash scene investigation.

Education Development Center. Teaching middle school students to be active researchers. (1999, September 1). Retrieved from http://www.edc.org/news room/articles/teaching_middle_school_students_be_active_researchers

This online article describes numerous approaches to increasing the accessibility of junior and high school science courses.

SciTrain Accessible Curriculum Strategies. Retrieved from http://www.catea .gatech.edu/scitrain

This Web site is funded through a grant from the National Science Foundation and administered by the Georgia Tech Center for Assistive Technology and Environmental Access (CATEA). It offers free online training to help teachers make their science, math, and computer science curriculum more accessible for students with disabilities. It offers resources on assistive technology as well as general strategies for adapting the curriculum.

Social Studies

StudyStack. Retrieved from http://www.studystack.com/About.jsp

This Web site allows students to review information in the form of online flashcards, discarding the cards they have learned and keeping the ones they still need to review. Each card can show multiple pieces of information, and the whole stack can be automatically sorted by any one of the pieces of information. The same information can be displayed as flashcards, a matching game, a word search puzzle, and a hangman game. Students can also export the data to a cell phone or PDA. They can use premade flashcards or design their own.

Autism

Autism Internet Modules (AIM). Retrieved from http://www.autisminternet modules.org
This site offers comprehensive information to assist those working and living with individuals with autism spectrum disorders (ASD) as they work to increase their knowledge and skills. AIM is working to develop 60 modules specific to autism, including topics such as assessment and identification, characteristics, evidence-based practices and interventions, transition to adulthood, and employment. The modules are free and site administrators are working to transcribe them into over five languages.

Tinsnips. Retrieved from http://www.tinsnips.org
This site provides a special education resource that strives to share a variety of specialized teaching tools, techniques, worksheets, and activities with teachers of students who have autism spectrum disorders and related developmental disabilities.

Zac Browser. Retrieved from http://www.zacbrowser.com
This site offers a free Web browser developed specifically for children with autism and autism spectrum disorders. The creators made the browser for their grandchild and share it. It contains games and activities specifically for kids with autism spectrum disorders. Note that using the browser disables the keyboard so that only the mouse works.

Vision

American Printing House for the Blind. Retrieved from http://www.aph.org/index.htm
This site contains numerous resources, from accessibility ideas to products.

Florida School for the Blind. Retrieved from http://www.fsdb.k12.fl.us
This site contains valuable resources for those who work with individuals who are blind. There are links under academics or outreach services for numerous resources and Web sites.

Learning Ally. Retrieved from http://www.learningally.org
This national nonprofit organization (formerly Recording for the Blind and Dyslexic or RFB&D) specializes in accessible educational materials for students with disabilities. The site contains accessible book titles available in every subject area and grade level, from kindergarten through graduate studies.

Learning through Listening. Retrieved from http://www.learningthrough listening.org

This Web site is designed for all educators in grades K–12 to support the use of audiobooks from Learning Ally. Users must register to access free, listening-focused content and skill-building exercises, such as lesson plans, classroom activities, teaching strategies, and listening resources.

Read the Words. Retrieved from http://www.readthewords.com

This site offers a free, online service that can read any text a user enters aloud, including Word files and PDFs as well as Internet sites. Users can choose from different voices, and the Spanish speakers read aloud in Spanish. Although users must register and create a profile, everything is free. The site launched in January 2008 with a goal to assist students with learning disabilities. Information users enter is stored in a personal profile and then can be downloaded for an iPod, Web site, blog, or podcast.

Texas School for the Blind and Visually Impaired. Retrieved from http://www.tsbvi.edu

This school's Web site includes information about instruction for children who are blind or visually impaired, including the National Agenda for Children and Youth Who Are Blind or Visually Impaired.

Hearing

National Center for Hearing Assistive Technology (NCHAT). Retrieved from http://www.hearingloss.org/learn/hat.asp

This agency promotes the use of technology to maximize the residual hearing of people who are hard of hearing. The Web site features information on cochlear implants, hearing aids, and other assistive technologies that benefit individuals with hearing impairment.

Technology Access Program (TAP). Retrieved from http://tap.gallaudet.edu

This project out of Gallaudet College conducts research related to communication technologies and services, with the goal of producing knowledge useful to industry, government, and deaf and hard-of-hearing consumers in the quest for equality in communications. This Web site includes information and numerous links about AT for hearing impairment. Information about current TAP projects, including the Rehabilitation Engineering and Research Center (RERC) on Telecommunications Access and the RERC on Hearing Enhancement and Assistive Devices, is also provided.

Communication

AAC Intervention. Retrieved from http://www.aacintervention.com

This Web site, created by Caroline Musselwhite and Julie Maro, has numerous AAC resources. Both the tip of the month and the activities pages offer excellent resources for individuals interested in AAC.

Askability. Retrieved from http://www.askability.org.uk/Default.aspx
This European Web site is presented entirely in symbols to enable children with learning disabilities to become informed about ongoing current affairs and also to create a central forum for children to express their views and opinions.

Assistive and Augmentative Communication (AAC) Parent Resources. Retrieved from http://www.circleofinclusion.org/english/augcomm/index.html
This Web site, designed by a parent of a young girl with cerebral palsy, contains numerous resources explaining what AAC is and providing ideas for implementation in numerous settings.

Augmentative and Alternative Communication (AAC) Connecting Young Kids (YAACK). Retrieved from http://aac.unl.edu/yaack/index.html
This Web site provides information and guidance and serves as a complete resource on many aspects of AAC with regard to young children.

Augmentative Communication, Inc. (ACI) Listserv. Retrieved from http://disabilities.temple.edu/programs/aac/acolug
Augmentative Communication Inc. (ACI) hosts a listserv to assist people who use AAC, as well as their friends and family.

Blackwell's Best. Retrieved from http://www.vickiblackwell.com
This Web site was created by a classroom teacher to provide ideas and resources to incorporate technology in the classroom.

Glass AAC Group On-Demand Training. Retrieved from http://sites.google.com/site/glassaacgroup/on-demand-training-2
This site contains numerous training options for specific devices and strategies relating to AAC. It is an extraordinary list of resources for those interested in training in AAC.

Pics4Learning. Retrieved from http://pics.tech4learning.com
This site contains a copyright-friendly image library for teachers and students. Images have been donated and permission has been granted for teachers and students to use all of the featured images.

Rehabilitation Engineering and Research Center on Augmentative/Alternative Communication (RERC-AAC). Retrieved from http://aac-rerc.psu.edu
The AAC-RERC, funded through the National Institute on Disability and Rehabilitation Research (NIDRR), is a collaborative organization conducting research, development, training, and dissemination activities aimed at assisting people with disabilities who rely on improve augmentative and alternative communication (AAC) technologies. The AAC-RERC advances and promotes AAC technologies and supports the individuals who use, manufacture, and recommend them.

Signing Savvy. Retrieved from http://www.signingsavvy.com
This site provides a searchable online sign language dictionary with video. The site contains high-resolution videos of American Sign Language (ASL) signs, finger-spelled words, and other common signs.

Speech-to-Speech (STS) Relay Services. Retrieved from http://www.fcc.gov/cgb/dro/sts.html
Within the United States, users can call a toll-free telephone number to access the service called Speech-to-Speech (STS) in their state. STS is a form of Relay Services that provides Communications Assistants (CAs) for people with speech disabilities who have difficulty being understood on the phone. STS CAs are trained individuals familiar with many different speech patterns and language-recognition skills. The CA makes the call and repeats the user's words exactly.

University of Buffalo AT Basics. Retrieved from http://atto.buffalo.edu/registered/ATBasics.php
This Web site contains the AT Basic Modules, which provide general assistive technology information on a variety of related uses for elementary students with disabilities. They include links to tutorials on the setup and use of several products as well as links to related resources.

University of Nebraska-Lincoln AAC Centers. Retrieved from http://aac.unl.edu
This site, available through the University of Nebraska-Lincoln, offers numerous augmentative and alternative communication (AAC) strategies that assist people with severe communication disabilities.

Wisconsin Assistive Technology Initiative (WATI). Retrieved from http://www.wati.org
This Web site contains numerous free resources on AT implementation and assessment. Curriculum modifications and forms can be easily downloaded and shared. The goal of WATI is to improve the outcomes and results for children with disabilities from birth to age 21 through the use of assistive technology to access services, curriculum, and school and community activities.

Early Childhood

Alliance for Technology Access. Retrieved from http://www.ataccess.org/index.php?option=com_content&view=article&id=37&Itemid=44
This site provides information on how to adapt toys for children with disabilities.

Center for Best Practices in Early Childhood Education. Retrieved from http://www.wiu.edu/thecenter

This site provides a list of articles regarding using technology with children in the classroom.

Let's Play! Project. Retrieved from http://letsplay.buffalo.edu
This site gives information about young children and play. It offers ideas about enhancing play opportunities for children with disabilities through the use of assistive technology, including assistance with positioning, mobility, communication, and toys.

Simplified Technology. Retrieved from http://www.lburkhart.com
Linda Burkart's site provides assistive technology Web and vendor resources. It also offers strategies for using augmentative communication with children with disabilities.

Access Issues/Motor

Better Living through Technology. Retrieved from http://www.bltt.org/quick tips/fao_onehandedtyping.htm
This site provides information on how to implement and teach one-handed typing, with ideas to speed input and access options. A free download is available to allow users to remap a standard computer keyboard with a layout designed for a one-handed user. Both right- and left-handed options are available.

Camera Mouse. Retrieved from http://www.cameramouse.org
Camera Mouse is a free head-tracking program for computer access.

Click-N-Type Virtual Keyboard. Retrieved from http://cnt.lakefolks.org
This site offers a free, online virtual keyboard, available in numerous languages. The software is designed to allow anyone with a disability that prevents him or her from typing on a physical computer keyboard to send keystrokes to virtually any Windows application by using a mouse, trackball, touch screen, or other pointing device.

Ohio State University Medical Center Patient Handouts. Retrieved from http://medicalcenter.osu.edu/patientcare/patient_education/Pages/index.aspx
The Ohio State University Medical Center provides information on particular illnesses and information about attaining a healthy lifestyle. Their resources include numerous positioning and exercise handouts. Click on exercise/rehabilitation handouts and find resources on everything from lower body to aquatic exercises. Handouts are printable to give to families.

Computers

BrowseAloud. Retrieved from http://www.browsealoud.com/page.asp?pg_id=80004

BrowseAloud is a free download for Mac and PC that will read Web sites aloud and highlight words as they are read.

Kaboose. Retrieved from http://resources.kaboose.com
This site offers both shareware and freeware for kids for the Mac and PC, categorized by age, subject, and activity.

Microsoft Accessibility. Retrieved from http://www.microsoft.com/enable
This site offers a guide to accessibility and accessible technology resources, as well as a number of tutorials to teach Microsoft computer products to individuals with different disabilities.

Northern Grid. Retrieved from http://www.northerngrid.org/ngflwebsite/sennew/start.html
This site is maintained by a nonprofit organization in Europe designed to support schools and local authorities to promote high standards in schools. The site has numerous special education resources, from software to switch access.

Trace Center. Retrieved from http://trace.wisc.edu/world/computer_access
This site offers links to shareware and freeware for adapting all types of computers, as well as guidelines, standards, operating system accessibility features, and information resources from the University of Wisconsin's Trace Center.

Switch Use

Bry-Back Manor. Retrieved from http://www.bry-backmanor.org/funstuff.html
This site contains downloadable games designed for young children with little or no reading skills. These games are designed for Macintosh and will not work on a PC or PC-compatible device.

Help Kidz Learn. Retrieved from http://www.helpkidzlearn.com
This Web site features free software and resources from Inclusive Technology. It includes interactive stories that are great for switch users.

Organizational/Time-Saving Strategies

del.icio.us. Retrieved from http://del.icio.us
This site allows users to store their favorite Web sites as bookmarks online, access the same bookmarks from any computer, and use tags to organize and remember bookmarks. This site is particularly useful for those who struggle to navigate the Internet.

Google Docs. Retrieved from http://www.google.com/google-d-s/tour1.html
This is a free, Web-based word processor and spreadsheet that allows users to share documents and collaborate online. It offers a way to store a document online, work on it from any computer, and give access to others as well.

Meeting Wizard. Retrieved from http://www.meetingwizard.com
This free Web site service enables users to plan and facilitate meetings by sending online invitations, proposing optional dates, managing responses, and sending automatic reminders.

Remember the Milk. Retrieved from http://www.rememberthemilk.com
This free, online service allows users to create and manage lists. There are lots of other helpful resources and features as well.

Rminder. Retrieved from http://www.rminder.com
This free, online resource allows users to enter information on a Web site in text and generate an automatic voice reminder message that is sent to a selected phone number at a specific time. This site also allows users to type in a message that it converts to a voice phone call to the number provided.

Ta-Da Lists. Retrieved from http://www.tadalist.com
This Web-based system allows users to create a to-do list online as well as view lists created by others who choose to share them.

Glossary of Key Terms

AAC   *See* Augmentative and Alternative Communication (AAC)

Abandonment   A situation that occurs when a person with a disability stops using an assistive technology device or service; on average, one-third of optional assistive technologies are abandoned, most within the first three months.

Activities of Daily Living (ADL)   A set of daily self-care tasks such as feeding, bathing, dressing, and grooming; the level of ability to perform ADL provides a measurement of an individual's degree of disability and functioning. ADL equipment, which is designed to make an individual more independent in a specific daily living task, includes bath seats, toileting aids, built-up spoon handles, and zipper pulls.

ADA   *See* Americans with Disabilities Act of 1990 (ADA)

ADL   *See* Activities of Daily Living (ADL)

Americans with Disabilities Act of 1990 (ADA)   This law clarified the civil rights of persons with disabilities and specified equal access to public places, employment, transportation, and telecommunications; employers are expected to provide "reasonable accommodations," and public and private entities that provides services (i.e., health care) are expected to make reasonable modifications, unless doing so would cause them undue hardship.

App   Short for application software, this type of user-driven computer software is designed to help people perform specific tasks.

Assistive Technology (AT)   Any item, piece of equipment, or system, whether acquired commercially, modified, or customized, that is commonly used to increase, maintain, or improve functional capabilities of individuals with disabilities. AT is a tool used by someone with a disability to perform everyday tasks, such as getting dressed, moving around, or controlling his or her environment, learning, working, or engaging in recreational activities.

Assistive Technology Services   Any service that directly assists an individual with a disability in the selection, acquisition, or use of an assistive technology device.

AT   *See* Assistive Technology (AT)

Augmentative and Alternative Communication (AAC)   Devices that can either augment or provide a voice for persons with severe expressive language impairments. *See also* Speech Generating Device (SGD)

CART   *See* Computer-Assisted Real-Time Translation (CART)

Computer-Assisted Real-Time Translation (CART)   An AT solution for persons with significant hearing impairments; it involves a specially trained typist or stenographer who captures what is being spoken and projects the text onto a display.

CPE   *See* Customer-Premises Equipment (CPE)

Customer-Premises Equipment (CPE)   Telecommunications equipment used in the home or office (or other premises) to originate, route, or terminate telecommunications.

Disability   A term that encompasses the complex interaction between an individual's physical, built, social, or attitudinal environment and his or her functional limitations from physical, sensory, communication, or cognitive impairments.

DME   *See* Durable Medical Equipment (DME)

Durable Medical Equipment (DME)   Assistive devices that serve a medical purpose; are able to withstand repeated use; are not useful to an individual in the absence of an illness, injury, functional impairment, or congenital abnormality; and are appropriate for use in or out of the patient's home.

EADL   *See* Electronic Aids to Daily Living (EADL)

Early Intervention (EI)   Educational programs that target children from birth to three years old and are designed to improve the children's developmental, social, and learning outcomes; such programs often include speech and language therapy, physical therapy, occupational therapy, social work, and assistive technology.

EARN   *See* Employer Assistance and Resource Network (EARN)

ECU   *See* Environmental Control Unit (ECU)

EI   *See* Early Intervention (EI)

Electronic Aids to Daily Living (EADL)   Technologies that provide alternative control of electrical devices within the environment and increase independence in tasks of daily living; within the home or work environments, EADLs can control audiovisual equipment, communication equipment, doors, electric beds, security equipment, lights, and appliances.

Employer Assistance and Resource Network (EARN)   A resource for employers seeking to recruit, hire, retain, and advance qualified employees with disabilities. EARN supports employers by providing confidential, no-cost consultation and technical assistance, customized training, comprehensive online resources, and links to state and local community-based organizations serving job seekers with disabilities.

Environmental Control Unit (ECU)   An alternative term for electronic aids to daily living (EADL) that is considered less accurate because it emphasizes the item being controlled (i.e., the telephone) rather than the task being aided (i.e., communication).

504 Plan   Offered under the Section 504 of the Rehabilitation Act, this education program is designed to accommodate school-age children who need accommodations or modifications in order to achieve academic success, but who do not need special education services.

Function   The physiological action or activity of a body part, organ, or system.

HTI   *See* Human Technology Interface (HTI)

Human Technology Interface (HTI)   The interaction between people and technological devices in their environment; individuals with impairments that affect this interaction may need special consideration in the design, function, or placement of the devices they want or need to activate.

ICF   *See* International Classification of Functioning, Disability, and Health (ICF)

IDEA   *See* Individuals with Disabilities Education Act of 1990 (IDEA)

IEP   *See* Individualized Education Program (IEP)

IFSP   *See* Individualized Family Service Plan (IFSP)

IPE   *See* Individualized Plan for Employment (IPE)

Impairment   A biomedical, underlying functional condition that is intrinsic to a person and constitutes the essential health component of disability; impairments may be sensory (difficulty in hearing, touch, or visual impairment), physical (difficulties in moving or standing up), cognitive or psychological (difficulty in coping with stress, depression, thinking and remembering).

Individualized Education Program (IEP)   Mandated by the Individuals with Disabilities Education Act (IDEA), the IEP documents and guides the process of identifying and referring eligible school-age children for special education services, assessing their needs, planning and implementing individualized programs to meet their needs, and monitoring and evaluating the programs' effectiveness; the IEP must indicate that AT has been considered as a way "to provide meaningful access to the general curriculum."

Individualized Family Service Plan (IFSP)   Mandated by the Individuals with Disabilities Education Act (IDEA), the IFSP documents and guides the early intervention (EI) process for young children with disabilities and their families, with the goal of improving the children's physical, cognitive, social, and emotional growth.

Individualized Plan for Employment (IPE)   A written document created by a state VR agency that outlines an individual's vocational goals and the services to be provided to help the individual reach those goals.

Individuals with Disabilities Education Act of 1990 (IDEA)   Also known as P.L. 101–476, this legislation specifies that AT devices and services be provided to children from birth to age 21 to facilitate education in a regular classroom if such devices and services are required as part of the student's special education, related services, or supplementary aids and services.

International Classification of Functioning, Disability, and Health (ICF)   Released in 2001 by the World Health Organization (WHO), this conceptual model of disability provides a common framework and language for the description of health and health-related domains; it views disability and functioning as outcomes of the interactions between health conditions and contextual factors.

JAN   *See* Job Accommodation Network (JAN)

Job Accommodation Network (JAN)   A free service that offers employers and individuals ideas about effective workplace accommodations; vocational counselors, employees, or employers can perform individualized searches for workplace accommodations based on a job's functional requirements, the functional limitations of the individual, environmental factors, and other pertinent information.

Least Restrictive Environment (LRE)   A mandate of the Individuals with Disabilities Education Act (IDEA) that requires children with disabilities to receive their special education in settings that provides access to their greatest participation in the regular classroom while ensuring maximum educational benefit.

LRE   *See* Least Restrictive Environment (LRE)

ODEP   *See* Office of Disability Employment Policy (ODEP)

Office of Disability Employment Policy (ODEP)   A sub-cabinet level agency in the U.S. Department of Labor that is charged with building collaborative partnerships and delivering authoritative and credible data to ensure that people with disabilities are fully integrated into the American workforce.

PAAT   *See* Protection and Advocacy for Assistive Technology (PAAT)

Prosthetic   A type of artificial device used to replace or augment a missing or impaired body part.

Protection and Advocacy for Assistive Technology (PAAT)   A federal program that provides funding to assist individuals with disabilities in the acquisition, utilization, or maintenance of assistive technology devices or services through case management, legal representation, and self-advocacy training.

Reasonable Accommodation   Any change in the work environment or in the way things are customarily done that enables an individual with a disability to apply for a job, perform a job, or gain equal access to the benefits and privileges of a job.

Rehabilitation Act of 1973   A U.S. law that authorizes and provides funding for rehabilitation programs and services, among them the state-federal vocational rehabilitation system, centers for independent living, and the National Institute on Disability and Rehabilitation Research. Section 504 of the act prohibits discrimination on the basis of disability in employment and in the delivery of services by state and private programs that receive federal funding.

Rehabilitation Engineering and Assistive Technology Society of North America (RESNA)   This organization hosts an academic credentialing program in assistive technology that offers national participation for three specialties: assistive technology professional (ATP); seating and mobility specialist (SMS); and rehabilitation engineering technologist (RET).

Rehabilitation Engineering Research Center for the Advancement of Cognitive Technologies (RERC-ACT) A government-funded scientific effort to develop assistive technologies focused on vocational and literacy skills, service provision, and enhanced caregiving supports for persons with significant cognitive impairments.

Rehabilitation Technology The use of technology, engineering, or scientific principles to meet the needs of and address the barriers faced by people with disabilities in areas which include education, rehabilitation, employment, transportation, independent living, and recreation; rehabilitation technology is divided into three categories: rehabilitation engineering, assistive technology devices, and assistive technology services.

Repetitive Strain or Stress Injuries (RSI) Injuries that occur when too much stress is placed on a part of the body, usually from repeating the same movements over and over, resulting in pain, inflammation, muscle strain, or tissue damage.

RERC-ACT *See* Rehabilitation Engineering Research Center for the Advancement of Cognitive Technologies (RERC-ACT)

RESNA *See* Rehabilitation Engineering and Assistive Technology Society of North America (RESNA)

Response to Intervention (RTI) A method of identifying and providing preliminary support to children with disabilities that incorporates assessment, intervention, and progress monitoring; RTI uses a multi-tiered, school-wide approach to promote student achievement and prevent behavior problems.

RSI *See* Repetitive Strain or Stress Injuries (RSI)

RTI *See* Response to Intervention (RTI)

Scanning The most common indirect selection method used by persons with significant motor impairments. A selection set is presented on a display and is sequentially scanned by a light or cursor on the device; the user chooses the desired item by pressing a switch.

Section 504   This section of the Rehabilitation Act of 1973 required programs, services, and entities that receive federal funding to make reasonable accommodations and promote accessibility for people with disabilities.

SGD   *See* Speech Generating Device (SGD)

Speech Generating Device (SGD)   An electronic augmentative/alternative communication system used to supplement or replace speech or writing for individuals with disabilities. *See also* Augmentative and Alternative Communication (AAC)

TDD   *See* Telephone Device for the Deaf (TDD)

Technology-Related Assistance for Individuals with Disabilities Act of 1988   Also known as P.L. 100–407, the Tech Act provided funding to develop statewide, consumer-responsive information and training programs designed to meet the assistive technology needs of individuals with disabilities of all ages.

TEDP   *See* Telecommunications Equipment Distribution Program (TEDP)

Telecommunications Act of 1996   Section 255 of this law requires telecommunications equipment manufacturers and service providers to make their products and services accessible to people with disabilities, as long as this access is readily achievable.

Telecommunications Equipment Distribution Program (TEDP)   Funded through a monthly surcharge on consumer telephone services, this program provides accessible telephone services for consumers with disabilities who struggle with using today's telecommunication equipment because of their disability.

Telephone Device for the Deaf (TDD)   An assistive technology device that allows hearing- and speech-impaired persons to communicate on the telephone by typing a text conversation; also known as a teletypewriter (TTY).

Teletypewriter (TTY)   An assistive technology device that allows hearing- and speech-impaired persons to communicate on the telephone by typing a text conversation; also known as a telephone device for the deaf (TDD).

TTY   *See* Teletypewriter (TTY)

Vocational Rehabilitation (VR)   Services designed to help individuals with disabilities gain or regain their independence through employment or some form of meaningful activity and reintegration into society; VR includes such services as vocational guidance, job training, occupational adjustment services, and job placement.

VR   *See* Vocational Rehabilitation (VR); Voice Recognition (VR)

Voice Recognition (VR)   A mass-market technology that offers computer access for many persons with motor impairment. Instead of using keyboard, VR users write or speak words out loud; the computer processor uses information from the user's individual voice file, compares it with digital models of words and phrases, and produces computer text.

Index

⑤SAGE researchmethods

The essential online tool for researchers from the world's leading methods publisher

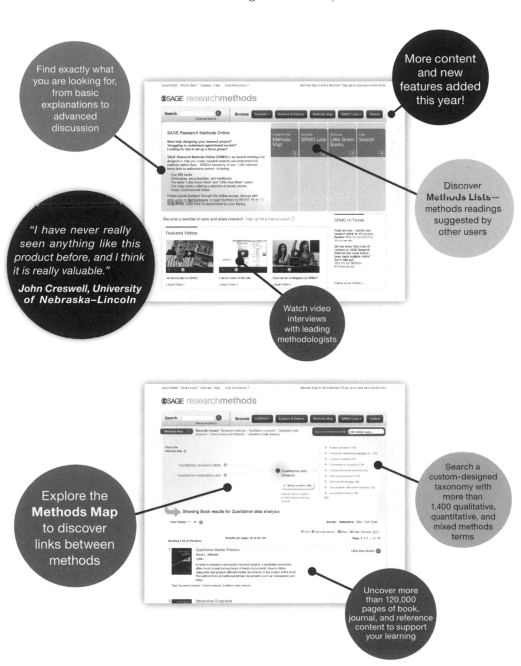

Find exactly what you are looking for, from basic explanations to advanced discussion

More content and new features added this year!

"I have never really seen anything like this product before, and I think it is really valuable."
John Creswell, University of Nebraska–Lincoln

Discover **Methods Lists**— methods readings suggested by other users

Watch video interviews with leading methodologists

Explore the **Methods Map** to discover links between methods

Search a custom-designed taxonomy with more than 1,400 qualitative, quantitative, and mixed methods terms

Uncover more than 120,000 pages of book, journal, and reference content to support your learning

Find out more at
www.sageresearchmethods.com